Working with Goals in Psychotherapy and Counselling

Working with Goals in Psychotherapy and Counselling

Edited by

Mick Cooper and Duncan Law

OXFORD
UNIVERSITY PRESS

OXFORD
UNIVERSITY PRESS

Great Clarendon Street, Oxford, OX2 6DP,
United Kingdom

Oxford University Press is a department of the University of Oxford.
It furthers the University's objective of excellence in research, scholarship,
and education by publishing worldwide. Oxford is a registered trade mark of
Oxford University Press in the UK and in certain other countries

First Edition published in 2018

Impression: 1

Published in the United States of America by Oxford University Press
198 Madison Avenue, New York, NY 10016, United States of America

British Library Cataloguing in Publication Data

Data available

Library of Congress Control Number: 2017959063

ISBN 978–0–19–879368–7

Printed and bound by
CPI Group (UK) Ltd, Croydon, CR0 4YY

Contents

List of contributors

Suzanne Byrne
Institute of Psychiatry, Psychology and Neuroscience, Kings College London, UK

Mick Cooper
Department of Psychology, University of Roehampton, UK

Windy Dryden
Goldsmiths University of London, UK

Julian Edbrooke-Childs
Anna Freud National Centre for Children and Families, UK

Amy Feltham
Common Room, UK

Nick Grey
Sussex Partnership NHS Foundation Trust, UK

Lydia Harris
Expert by Experience, UK

Daniel Hayes
Evidence Based Practice Unit, UCL and Anna Freud National Centre for Children and Families, UK

Jenna Jacob
Child Outcomes Research Consortium (CORC), UK

Duncan Law
Anna Freud National Centre for Children and Families, and MindMonkey Associates, UK

Roslyn Law
Anna Freud National Centre for Children and Families, UK

Christopher Lloyd
London Metropolitan University, UK

Thomas Mackrill
Institute for Social Work, Metropolitan University College, Frederiksberg, Denmark

Kate Martin
Common Room, UK

John McLeod
Department of Psychology, Faculty of Social Sciences, The University of Oslo, Norway

Aaron Sefi
XenZone, UK

Avi Shmueli
University College London, UK

Peter Stratton
University of Leeds, UK

Tracey Taylor
Centre for Anxiety Disorders & Trauma, South London & Maudley NHS Foundation Trust, UK

Cathy Troupp
Eating Disorders Service, Great Ormond Street Hospital, UK

Georgiana Shick Tryon
The Graduate Center of the City University of New York, USA

Leanne Walker
Expert by Experience, UK

Isabelle Whelan
Evidence Based Practice Unit, UCL
and Anna Freud National Centre for
Children and Families, UK

Miranda Wolpert
Evidence Based Practice Unit, UCL
and Anna Freud National Centre for
Children and Families, UK

Chapter 1

Introduction

Mick Cooper and Duncan Law

The goals of this chapter are to:

- ◆ Present the rationale for developing this book.
- ◆ Define goals and key goal-related terms.
- ◆ Discuss the development of working with goals in counselling and psychotherapy.
- ◆ Review the arguments for working with goals.
- ◆ Review the challenges and limitations of working with goals.
- ◆ Outline the style and structure of the book.

Gita is a 42-year-old woman who seeks therapy after a divorce. In her first meeting with her therapist, Sonia, she speaks of her overwhelming feeling since her divorce three years ago. She feels she cannot live with the feelings that range from despair to anxiety through guilt and shame. Sonia listens to her story patiently and with humanity. Gita is distressed by the telling and feels she will burst with the strength of her feelings, but she tells her story, spurred on by the interest and compassion of her listener. After a while, Sonia gently enquires about her hopes for engaging in therapy. Gita is unsure—she knows she does not want to feel as she does but cannot see beyond the emotions, she wants them gone. Over the next two sessions, Sonia listens to more of Gita's story of her life and her divorce. Together, they begin to construct a shared narrative that weaves together Gita's life story, recent events, and the strong thoughts and feelings she experiences. They begin, tentatively, to shape ideas together about what they might helpfully focus on. Gita wants to find a way of moving on: she wants to get past her feelings of loss, and she wants to prepare herself for thinking about a new relationship. This shaping moves the narrative from what has been to what could be—it shifts from the unbearable past to the hoped-for future.

Gita and Sonia work together, moving from listening to shaping to listening—constructing and refining. Eventually they have a shared understanding and agreement of what the forthcoming work should be—they write the agreement down. Gita feels listened to and understood, she feels that Sonia is on her side and they have a shared idea of the direction of travel. Gita goes on to rate how far away she feels from getting to where she wants to be. She and Sonia revisit these ratings from time to time during the therapy to help them both see the progress that has been made and the distance still to travel. Over a number of sessions, the unbearable feelings begin to subside and after further sessions still Gita rates her progress as being well down the line to her goals. Although she has still a way to go, she feels the therapy has helped her far enough down the road to continue to make progress on her own for now. Gita decides to bring therapy to an end, and continues on her journey of self-development. When things get difficult and the feelings re-emerge, she is able to think back to the therapy and remember the ratings she made to remind herself how far she has already come. This helps her carry on with her progress towards her goals.

Gita's journey exemplifies what it means to work with goals in counselling and psychotherapy. It is a complex, subtle, and dialogical process, in which collaboratively-agreed goals can provide focus and direction to the therapeutic work. Gita's goals give her hope, and also a sense of direction and purpose. They support Gita to move towards her future.

Terminology

According to the *Online Etymology Dictionary*, the word 'goal' emerged in the sixteenth century, referring to the endpoint of a race. Its origins are uncertain, but may be related to the Old English *gal, meaning 'obstacle' or 'barrier'. In the contemporary psychological literature, probably the most widely used definition of goals comes from Austin and Vancouver (1996): 'internal representations of desired states' (p. 338). A more recent and nuanced definition, also used widely in the psychological field, comes from Kruglanski (2009): 'subjectively desirable states of affairs that the individual intends to attain through action' (p. 29). This is similar to Elliot and Niesta's (2009) definition, 'a cognitive representation of a future object that an organism is committed to approach or avoid' (p. 58).

Across these definitions, several inter-related features of goals are posited. First, goals are a mental phenomenon—they are not, for instance, behaviours or physiological responses, per se. However, we can refer to 'goal-directed activities', or 'goal processes' as descriptions of the behaviours associated with goals. Second, closely related to this, goals are conceptions, cognitions, or representations, rather than the thing in itself. Third, however, goals are always oriented towards an object: the goal object. This may be a state of affairs, an entity, an event, an experience, or a particular characteristic. Fourth, goals have a motivational element. They are, as Elliot and Niesta (2009) write, 'inherently valenced': a distinctively 'hot' form of cognitive representation. Goals matter to the person, they are affect-laded. Fifth, goals are about the future. They describe what the person wants to happen in the coming hours, days, or years. Finally, goals are aspirations that the person sets for themselves. This distinguishes them, for instance, from 'hopes' or 'expectations', which a person may be able to attain through others' actions.

In recent years, within the psychological and psychotherapeutic literature, several other concepts have been proposed and researched, which share many of these characteristics of goals. These include 'personal projects' (e.g. Little, Salmela-Aro, & Phillips, 2007), 'personal strivings' (e.g. Emmons, 1986), 'possible selves' (Markus & Nurius, 1986), 'personal concerns' (Cox & Klinger, 2002), 'wants' (Cooper, 2012), and 'aims' (Emanuel, 2013). In addition, the English language contains several other terms that share many of the properties of goals: for instance, 'desires', 'intentions', 'purposes', 'objectives', 'wants', and 'wishes'.

Although these terms refer to similar phenomena, there are subtle and important differences among them. For instance, a 'purpose', in contrast to an 'aim', is a desire that is embedded in a higher level system of personal meanings; and an 'objective' is likely to be more conscious than a 'desire'. What is relatively distinctive about a 'goal'—compared, for instance, with a 'purpose' or a 'personal striving'—is that it has a particularly clear, specific, and well-defined object. We might say, for instance, 'My goal is to drink three bottles of water today'; but we would be less likely to describe this as a personal striving. With such terms, the object of our desires tends to be more diffuse, and there is more of a focus on the journey towards it. Goals, in contrast to wants or desires, also have a specific commitment to act.

Throughout this book, we will use the word 'goals' to describe a desired state of affairs that we intend to attain, as it is the most commonly used term in both the psychological and psychotherapeutic literature. However, as above, we acknowledge that the term can imply a relatively fixed and definite endpoint, and want to emphasize that we are not necessarily using it in this way. That is, by 'goal', we mean something that we are striving for in the future. This may include a highly diffuse, complex, and unconscious 'endpoint'; as well as more focused, defined, and conscious objectives.

In working with goals within counselling and psychotherapy, we can also distinguish among several goal-related concepts and processes. *Goal-setting* is the process of identifying and establishing goals—generally at the start of therapy, although they may be re-set further on in the process. *Goal-tracking* (or goal-monitoring) is the evaluation of clients' progress towards their goals, generally through some kind of individualized outcome measure. *Goal-discussion*, or metatherapeutic communication about goals, refers to any process in which client and therapist collaboratively talk about the goals for therapy. *Goal-oriented therapy* encompasses these concepts, and refers to a therapeutic approach in which the setting, tracking, and discussion of clients' goals forms a central element of the therapeutic work. *Goal-agreement*, derived from the psychotherapy research literature, is the extent to which therapists and clients are matched in their understandings of the objectives for therapy. Goal-oriented therapies generally aim towards high levels of goal-agreement, but the two dimensions are not necessarily synonymous. Finally, *goal-based formulations* refer to understandings of clients and their problems that are based on a teleological, purpose-oriented understanding of self (for instance, 'plan analysis', see Chapter 3, this volume). Goal-based formulations may be carried out within a goal-oriented therapy, but the two processes are not necessarily synonymous. For instance, a meaning-centred therapist might understand a client's difficulties in terms of purposelessness, but they might not actually set goals for the therapeutic work.

Development and scope of goal-oriented practices

Early psychoanalysis focused on behaviours that were driven by instincts unknown (and, to an extent, unknowable) to the client (e.g. Freud, 1900). Here, where desires were driven by unconscious mechanisms, direct enquiry into client goals had little value (see Chapter 9, this volume). In the mid-twentieth century, Charlotte Buhler (1962) is credited as being the first to argue for a more explicit link between the life goals of the client and the goals of therapy (Michalak & Grosse Holtforth, 2006). This gave legitimacy to a therapist enquiring about a client's goals, but explicit goal-setting for the therapeutic work remained firmly professionally led. Over the coming years there was a growing interest in hearing what people wanted to get from therapy as part of the focus of the work itself. This interest became incorporated across a range of emerging modalities, notably cognitive therapy (Beck, 1979). Arguably, however, it was not until the work of the brief solution-focused therapy movement in the later part of the twentieth century—with interest in helping clients reach their 'preferred futures' (de Shazer, 1991)—that client goals took centre stage and were endorsed as the primary focus of therapeutic work. This stance has courted controversy and influence over modern psychological therapies ever since (see Chapter 9, this volume). It has also taken a prominent role in other psychological practices that seek to facilitate individual development, such as coaching and consultation.

The ideas that underpin the use of goals in psychotherapy and counselling have not developed along a linear trajectory. Rather, research evidence and theory have developed from the interplay of a range of interconnecting disciplines. In recent times the influences have mainly been derived from:

- experimental and theoretical psychology—particularly the field of goal-oriented behaviours and motivation (Austin & Vancouver, 1996; Moskowitz & Grant, 2009; Chapter 3, this volume);

- philosophy—notably ideas around 'agency' (Smith, 2015; and Chapter 2, this volume);

- medico-legal ethics—particularly relating to issues around informed consent (Fisher & Oransky, 2008, Department of Health, 2009; Chapters 2 and 8, this volume).

These constructs have, in turn, been shaped within in the field of psychotherapy and counselling by practitioners themselves, testing and developing them through:

- applied goal-oriented practice—developing and sharing practice-based skills in using goals in therapy (Chapters 7, 8, and 9, this volume);

- applied research evidence—the scientific testing of common factors in therapy as well as modality-specific efficacy of practice (Duncan et al., 2010, Weisz & Kazdin, 2010; Roth & Fonagy, 2005; Chapter 5, this volume).

Both of these processes have brought into sharp focus the need to—and challenges of—measuring and monitoring clients' goals in therapy (Edbrooke-Childs, 2015, Chapter 6, this volume).

More recently still, people who use counselling and psychotherapy services have, themselves, begun to influence practice. This welcome increase in the power of service users' voices has led to service users rightly demanding more influence in decisions about their care. That is, to have greater say over the interventions they are involved in and how these take into account their unique contexts, goals, and wishes (see Chapter 4, this volume).

How these constructs and ideas have shaped practice has varied across the diversity of psychotherapy and counselling orientations. The reasons for these differences can, in part, be explained by the different settings in which the therapies tend to be applied. Cognitive-behavioural therapies, for instance, which are often delivered within a NHS-context, have had to develop a strong goal-focused approach because of the limited time periods that tend to be available. However, the cultures, histories, psychologies, and philosophical assumptions of each orientation have also shaped their attitudes towards working with goals (see Chapter 9, this volume). The humanistic therapy emphasis on 'being' over 'doing', for instance, has led to a wariness of goal-oriented work.

In England, recent policy has supported the use of goals in therapy. Implicitly, this has been through the 'recovery' and 'choice' agendas enshrined in the 'five year forward views' for the National Health Service (NHS), NHS England (2014), and Mental Health services, specifically The Mental Health Taskforce (2016) and more explicitly in 'consent to treatment' policy (Department of Health, 2009). In children's services, support for the use and monitoring of goals is set out in *Future in Mind* (NHS England & Department of Health, 2015).

Rationale for working with goals in counselling and psychotherapy

So why should therapists work with goals in counselling and psychotherapy? Clinically, as we saw in the work with Gita, goals may help focus and direct clients' and therapists' attention in the therapeutic work. This may be of particular importance in short-term work and in times of austerity, in which clients and therapists need to provide the most effective interventions with the least use of resources. Setting goals for therapy may also engender hope, help to energize clients towards their goals, enhance persistence, and help clients to find more effective strategies for achieving these goals. Through discussing and setting goals, clients may also develop a deeper insight into what it is that they really want in life: a crucial first step towards being able to get there. These potential benefits are supported by research from the psychology field, which suggests that people are more likely to achieve the things that they want if they set explicit goals (of a certain type, see Chapter 3, this volume). In addition, research shows that goal-agreement between therapist and client tends to be associated with better clinical outcomes (see Chapter 5, this volume).

There are also ethical arguments for working with goals in counselling and psychotherapy. As suggested above, a goal-oriented practice has the potential to be empowering for clients. Therapists—however 'client-centred' they are—will always have particular wants, hopes, or expectations in the therapeutic work. A goal-oriented approach puts the client's own, explicitly stated agenda at the heart of the therapeutic process. Orienting the work around the client's goals also means that the client's individualized wants take precedence over any diagnosis-based treatment plan. Research shows that clients with similar diagnoses can have very different objectives for therapy (e.g. Holtforth & Grawe, 2002). Clients who are depressed, for instance, may want to improve their interpersonal relationships, or develop strategies for becoming more active, or come to terms with childhood events. Different orientations make different assumptions about what such clients 'really' need, but a goal-oriented approach cuts underneath this and starts with the client's individually stated wants.

A goal-oriented approach also may be empowering to clients because it 'constructs' them as agentic choice-making beings, who have the possibility to act upon their worlds. Here, clients are not engaged with as victims of their circumstances or as passive 'sponges', but as people who have the potential to act towards—and achieve—their desired futures. By asking clients about their goals for therapy, counsellors or psychotherapists are implicitly communicating to clients that they respect their opinions and understandings.

Setting and discussing goals for therapy also may be empowering to clients because it can establish greater transparency in the therapeutic work. As suggested above, therapists—as well as clients—will always have things that they want from the therapeutic work, whether consciously or unconsciously held. A therapist, for instance, may want a client to 'feel more accepting of who he or she is', while a client may just want 'the pain to go away'. Not talking about these wants does not make them go away. Rather, it means that they can lie, unspoken, in the therapeutic work; and potentially lead to ruptures with clients and therapists pulling in different directions. Explicit goal-discussion, then, can bring these wants to the surface, and help to create a more open, trusting, and honest relationship.

Closely linked to the issue of empowerment, another strong argument for using goals in therapy is because this is what many clients want. Research suggests that around six out of ten laypeople want specific goals to be set in therapy, with around two out of ten not wanting this, and two out of ten not minding (Cooper & Norcross, 2015). The fact that mental health practitioners, when thinking about their own preferences as clients, are significantly less likely to want goals (with around four out of ten expressing a preference for this), suggests that therapists should be particularly wary of assuming that their clients have the same preferences as themselves.

Challenges to working with goals in counselling and psychotherapy

So, if working with goals in counselling and psychotherapy can be empowering to clients, is what many clients want, and can improve outcomes, why is it that many counsellors and psychotherapists are sceptical or even rejecting of this practice—particularly those of psychodynamic and humanistic orientations?

From a 'depth psychology' perspective—which holds that the principal determinants of human experience exist beneath the threshold of consciousness—perhaps the greatest limitation of a goal-oriented approach, as introduced above, is that it may be seen as focusing only on the most surface-level needs and wants of the client. That is, what clients are consciously aware of wanting—particularly at the start of therapy (for instance, 'to be happier') —may have little to do with their actual, unconscious needs and desires (for instance, 'to punish the world for not seeing my specialness'). Closely related to this, it can be argued that the goals that clients are willing to share with their therapists may be heavily 'censored', and not reflect their more destructive, 'unacceptable' impulses. In addition, from many therapeutic perspectives, what clients want—even at the most unconscious level—is not necessarily what they need. The client, for instance, who wants the world to see their specialness, may actually need to come to terms with their ordinariness to function effectively. From these perspectives, then, a goal-oriented therapy may not only miss clients' most significant therapeutic needs, but actually divert the therapy away from them.

For therapies that emphasize the healing potential of non-judgemental acceptance (such as person-centred and humanistic therapies, see Chapter 9, this volume), there can also be a concern that goal-oriented practice reinforces a process of self-evaluation and self-judgement (Rowan, 2008). From these perspectives, therapy works by helping clients come to accept all the different aspects of themselves. Here, goals may be seen as re-introducing concepts of success and failure, and leading clients to feel that they must be a certain way. From these perspectives, goals can also be seen as emphasizing attainment, striving, and doing over a more 'authentic' state of being; the future over the present. In other words, therapy becomes just one more domain in which clients must strive to achieve something, rather than having the opportunity to experience the fluidity and flow of here-and-now being. Indeed, to the extent that goal-striving is seen as the core sickness of a contemporary, Western, neo-liberal society—and meditative, Eastern *wu wei* ('non-doing') its remedy—a goal-oriented approach may be considered the very anathema of therapeutic healing.

There are also practical challenges to the process of working with goals in therapy. One that is commonly posited is that, in many instances, clients may not know what their goals are—so what is the point of asking them. Another challenge that is often raised is that clients' goals may change and evolve through the therapeutic process, particularly as clients become more aware of their deeper needs. Hence, goals that are set early on in therapy may actually become a barrier towards the therapeutic growth process.

To some extent, these divisions in attitudes towards goal-oriented practice emerge from differing psychological and philosophical assumptions. In particular, as we have seen above, those therapies that emphasize unconscious processes are less likely to attend to clients' verbally articulated goals, compared with those therapies that emphasize conscious processes (such as solution-focused therapy). In addition, therapies which consider reflective 'being' a more salutogenic (i.e. wellbeing enhancing) state than striving and 'doing', may be less likely to adopt a goal-oriented approach.

In many instances, however, the challenges to a goal-oriented therapy may be based on a relatively one-dimensional caricaturing of such practice. Hypothetically, a therapist who calls themselves 'goal-oriented' might fixate the work around particular goals, refuse to let clients modify them—whatever else transpires—and chastize their clients if they fail to achieve their objectives. However, this would be no more representative of a genuine goal-oriented practice than, for instance, the parroting of each client utterance would be representative of person-centred therapy. In reality, as we saw with Gita and Sonia, goal-oriented therapy is a complex, multifaceted, and nuanced endeavour, in which the therapeutic goals may be articulated and re-articulated multiple times. Here, the therapist is not treating the client's goals as fixed and definitive endpoints for therapy—which must be achieved at any costs—but as fluid, changeable, and, inevitably, approximate indicators of the client's preferred 'direction of travel'. In this respect, a client's goals are less like the final destination of a sea voyage, and more like the stars in the sky or the moon, which can provide orientation, guidance, and some illumination to the therapeutic work.

About this book

The aims of this book are to develop—and communicate—an understanding of how goals can be used in therapeutic practice. Our general assumption, as laid out above, is that goals have the potential to be a useful part of the therapeutic process, but there is a need to understand much more about how, when, and where they might be most helpful. In particular, some of the questions that we hope we can address through writing this book are:

- What are the different ways in which goals can be used in therapy?
- What can we learn from psychological theory and research about goals and how they can be used in practice?
- What kinds of goals may be most helpful in the therapeutic work?
- What is the relationship among goals, goal-agreement, and therapeutic outcomes?
- What are the best methods for setting goals?
- What are the best methods for tracking goals in therapy?
- How do different orientations view working with goals, and what can they contribute to a goal-oriented practice?

In this book, we also aim to address some of the challenges posed towards a goal-oriented perspective, as discussed above. For instance, how can goals be incorporated into a depth psychotherapeutic approach, and how can we work with goals in a flexible and responsive way? Here, as with all the questions above, we are not aiming to provide definitive answers. Rather, like the stars and the moon described above, we hope to present some illumination and guidance as we journey towards more effective, ethical, and client-oriented therapeutic practices.

In developing this book, we have very consciously oriented it towards readers from a range of orientations. Although, as discussed above, different approaches may be more or less positive towards goal-oriented work, we hope readers from all backgrounds will find ideas and practices here that are of use to their therapeutic work. Quite uniquely, in this book, we have also tried to ensure that the chapters are aimed at both adult and child practitioners. However, the focus is primarily on one-to-one work rather than working in groups, and we have not covered goal-oriented practices in the field of coaching or consultancy.

In an attempt to make the book accessible to a range of disciplines and experiences, we have given thought to the language used. Every discipline develops a language of its own with words that take on specific technical meaning. This is no less true in the field of counselling and psychotherapy as it is in any other profession. At best this technical language can help bring clarity of thought and precision of meaning to abstract and complex ideas. Precise definitions can bring a useful shorthand to discussion and can bring practitioners together in a shared understanding that can help develop thinking and practice. However, there is a downside to attempts at such semantic precision: within the different disciplines and sub-genres of the therapy professions words and phrases can take on such specific meaning as to create division rather than unity and collaboration. Indeed the title of this volume with its use of the words 'goals', 'psychotherapy', and 'counselling', could be argued to be some of the more controversial terms in the field.

Clearly language is important, and we have been cognizant in our use of it and in steering contributors to be mindful of their use too. However, we wished to avoid, as far as possible, getting too tied up in semantic knots by accepting broad definition terms—as with 'goals', above—and not to dictate to contributors use of technical language in very narrow ways. For example, 'client' is generally used throughout the book to be interchangeable with 'service user' or 'patient', which, in turn, is interchangeable shorthand for 'person who has an issue and chooses to work with a counsellor or therapist for whatever reason'. Of course, none of which quite capture the complexity of real people and real lives but all, we hope, serve as reasonable and respectful shorthand. Similarly, 'psychotherapy and counselling' are used interchangeably throughout this volume within the broad definition of 'talking therapies'. Talking therapies also include what others may prefer to label 'psychological therapies', 'psychological interventions', or for the very shorthand just 'therapy'.

In terms of structure, following this introduction, the book looks at the philosophical foundations of a goal-oriented approach to therapy (Chapter 2). It then considers the psychological evidence that can inform a goal-oriented practice (Chapter 3). Very importantly, we then consider how service users may consider the use of goals (Chapter 4). Chapter 5 reviews the evidence on the relationship between goals agreement and outcomes; and this leads into Chapter 6, which focuses on the tools that are available to measure and monitor goals. Chapters 7 and 8 focus more specifically on practice, with the former providing guidance on goal-setting, and the latter looking at work with goals across the therapeutic process. Finally, Chapter 9 considers goal-oriented practice from a range of therapeutic orientations, and looks at what they can contribute to the development of goal-oriented work.

Conclusion

This book brings together a range of ideas across the common theme of goals in psychotherapy and counselling. This is a purposeful attempt to further the debate around the value and efficacy of goals—and there is debate to be had. The diversity across psychotherapy theory and practice is testament to the richness of thinking within the field. We hope this volume adds informed ideas to the debate and, more importantly, we hope it adds to the knowledge of the efficacy that underlies the use of goals in practice. It is only through sound debate built on sound evidence that psychotherapy and counselling will continue the trajectory from practice built on tradition and belief to one of practice built on research, evidence, and critical inquiry.

Points for reflection

- What is your current attitude towards working with goals in counselling and psychotherapy?
- How helpful do you feel working with goals is in your own practice?
- What do you hope to gain from reading this book: what are your goals for reading it?

You may want to reflect on these questions now, and then again at the end of your engagement with this book.

References

Austin, J. T., & Vancouver, J. B. (1996). Goal constructs in psychology: Structure, process, and content. *Psychological Bulletin, 120*(3), 338–75. doi: 10.1037/0033-2909.120.3.338

Beck, A.T. (1979). *Cognitive therapy*. New York: Guilford Press.

Buhler, C. (1962). Goals of life and therapy. *American Journal of Psychoanalyis, 22*, 153–75.

Cooper, M. (2012). *A hierarchy of wants: Towards an integrative framework for counselling, psychotherapy and social change*. University of Strathclyde. Glasgow. Retrieved from pure.strath.ac.uk/portal

Cooper, M., & Norcross, J. C. (2015). *Mental health professionals and service users' preferences for therapy* [Unpublished dataset].

Cox, W. M., & Klinger, E. (2002). Motivational structure: Relationships with substance use and processes of change. *Addictive Behaviors, 27*(6), 925–40. doi: 10.1016/S0306-4603(02)00290-3

Department of Health (2009) Reference guide to consent for examination or treatment, 2nd Edition. London: Department of Health.

de Shazer, S. D. (1991). Putting Difference to Work. New York: Norton.

Duncan, B. L., Miller, S. D., Wampold, B. E., & Hubble, M. A. (2010). *The heart and soul of change: Delivering what works in therapy*. Washington D.C.: American Psychological Association.

Edbrooke-Childs, J., Jacob, J., Law, D., Deighton, J., & Wolpert, M. (2015). Interpreting standardized and idiographic outcome measures in CAMHS: what does change mean and how does it relate to functioning and experience? *Child and Adolescent Mental Health, 20*(3), 142–8.

Emanuel, R., Catty, J., Anscombe, E., Cantle, A., & Muller, H. (2014). Implementing an aim-based outcome measure in a psychoanalytic child psychotherapy service: Insights, experiences and evidence. *Clinical Child Psychology and Psychiatry, 19*(2), 169–83. doi: 1359104513485081.

Elliot, A. J., & Niesta, D. (2009). Goals in the context of the hierarchical model of approach-avoidance motivation. In G. B. Moskowitz & H. Grant (Eds.), *The Psychology of Goals* (pp. 56–76). New York: Guilford Press.

Emmons, R. A. (1986). Personal strivings: An approach to personality and subjective well-being. *Journal of Personality and Social Psychology, 51*(5), 1058–68. doi: 10.1037/0022-3514.51.5.1058

Fisher, C. B., & Oransky, M. (2008). Informed consent to psychotherapy: Protecting the dignity and respecting the autonomy of patients. *Journal of Clinical Psychology, 64*(5), 576–88.

Freud, S. (1900). *The Interpretation of Dreams*. Standard Edition, 4–5. Vintage: London.

Holtforth, M. G., & Grawe, K. (2002). Bern inventory of treatment goals: Part 1. Development and first application of a taxonomy of treatment goal themes. *Psychotherapy Research, 12*(1), 79–99.

Kruglanski, A. W., & Kopetz, C. (2009). What is so special (and nonspecial) about goals?: A view from the cognitive perspective. In G. B. Moskowitz & H. Grant (Eds.), *The Psychology of Goals* (pp. 27–55). New York: Guilford Press.

Little, B. R., Salmela-Aro, K., & Phillips, S. D. (Eds.). (2007). *Personal project pursuit: Goals, action, and human flourishing*. Mahwah, NJ: Lawrence Erlbaum Associates Publishers.

Markus, H., & Nurius, P. (1986). Possible selves. *American Psychologist, 41*(9), 954–69. doi: 10.1037/0003-066x.41.9.954

Mental Health Taskforce. (2016). *The five year forward view for mental health.*

Michalak, J., & Holtforth, M. G. (2006). Where do we go from here? The goal perspective in psychotherapy. *Clinical Psychology: Science and Practice, 13*(4), 346–65.

Moskowitz, G. B., & Grant, H. (Eds.). (2009). *The Psychology of Goals.* New York: Guilford Press.

NHS England. (2014). Five Year Forward View.

Roth, A., & Fonagy, P. (2005). *What works for whom?: a critical review of psychotherapy research.* 2nd Edition. New York: Guilford Press.

Rowan, J. (2008). Goals. *BACP North London Magazine* (59), 7.

Smith, R. (2015). Agency: A historical perspective. In *Constraints of Agency* (pp. 3–29). Springer International Publishing.

Weisz, J. R., & Kazdin, A. E. (Eds.). (2010). *Evidence-based psychotherapies for children and adolescents.* Guilford Press.

Chapter 2

Philosophical, conceptual, and ethical perspectives on working with goals in therapy

John McLeod and Thomas Mackrill

The goals of this chapter are:

♦ to identify and explore philosophical perspectives on the nature of human goals;

♦ to examine the relevance of these ways of understanding for the practice of goal-informed therapy;

♦ to develop a critical perspective on contemporary theory and research into therapeutic goals.

Introduction

Awareness and elucidation of client goals forms part of the work of counsellors, psychotherapists, and practitioners in fields such as life coaching and career counselling, where clients voluntarily initiate help-seeking. In some settings, client goals are formally recorded in a written contract or goal attainment form. In other therapy contexts, informal or implicit goal agreement emerges through the process of the work. Although therapy approaches differ in the degree to which they are explicitly goal-oriented, an awareness of the client's purpose or goal is ever-present. But what do we mean when we talk about 'goals'? How do we make sense of this concept? What are the moral and ethical dimensions of working with goals? This chapter considers some possible answers to these questions, and explores the implications of these positions for therapy practice.

The chapter does not claim to offer a comprehensive analysis of conceptual and ethical issues associated with the concept of a 'goal'. Rather, some key aspects of this topic are explored, as a means of encouraging readers to reflect on their own practice.

Explaining human action and behaviour

An important starting point, for any discussion of the concept of 'goal' is to acknowledge the extent to which this construct represents a radical break with a traditional scientific perspective. Modern science is based on an understanding of causality that assumes that an event is caused by some kind of force or disturbance that precedes it in time. For example, the river is flooding because it rained two days ago, and it rained two days ago because a weather front came in from the Atlantic ... and so on. We would not consider a statement such as 'it flooded because the water in the loch wanted to get to the sea' to be a scientific statement. The latter type of formulation can be described as *teleological*—an explanation that invokes a final cause. It is easy to see that teleological explanations are not consistent with what we generally regard as being a scientific approach.

Why is this important? It matters because the theories of therapy that we use are almost entirely organized around causal mechanisms: childhood experience leads to adult problems, therapist empathy facilitates a process of client change, negative automatic thoughts contribute to depression. In practice, therapists make sense of client problems, and the nature of effective interventions, using sophisticated ideas around different types of causality (see, e.g., Haynes, O'Brien, Kaholokula, & Witteman, 2012). Nevertheless, in the end all of this comes back to the simple idea that change occurs because a prior event causes a subsequent event. The notion that a therapy outcome could be in some sense caused by a later event (he became less depressed because he resolutely pursued his new goal of learning to sing/building a house/going to church) does not readily come across as offering a scientific basis for making sense of practice.

Philosopher Søren Kierkegaard (1843/1938) offers an understanding of why counsellors and indeed all human beings search for behavioural causes in the past, while he also emphasizes that such a perspective will always be insufficient. He wrote that:

> It is perfectly true, as philosophers say, that life must be understood backwards. But they forget the other proposition, that it must be lived forwards. And if one thinks over that proposition it becomes more and more evident that life can never really be understood in time because at no particular moment can I find the necessary resting place from which to understand it—backwards. (p. 18)

Although we typically understand our lives by looking to the past, we cannot conduct our lives if our attention is solely focused on the past. Orientation toward the future and having goals and a sense of purpose is necessary. Psychology and psychiatry tend to focus on the causes of behaviours, while psychotherapy which focuses on change, cannot really operate without a concept that grasps direction towards the future.

What is being suggested here is that, even though working with client goals is self-evidently a sensible and valuable thing to do, it represents a significant departure from any of the main theoretical frameworks that guide therapy practice. The significance, and necessity, of what might be described as 'goals talk' is that it reflects a taken-for-granted common-sense way of understanding that permeates everyday life. Human beings generally view themselves as purposeful, intentional beings who accept personal responsibility for their actions.

While the concept of *free* will is problematic for many individuals, and within many religious systems (e.g. karma), as well as from a scientific world-view, notions of *willingness* and *choice* are a lot easier to accommodate. Yes, our choices are constrained and determined in many respects, but at the same time we know that we are willing to do some things and not willing to do others.

The notion that to be human is to act with intentionality and with awareness of a lived future has been central to the phenomenological and existential tradition in philosophy (Brentano, 1973; Heidegger, 2010; Moran, 2000). From an existential perspective, wellbeing is related to having a clear sense of one's purpose and the future (Frankl, 1984). The ideas of the philosopher John Macmurray (1961), who influenced many contemporary psychologists, emphasized personal agency as an essential attribute of being human. For Macmurray, agency is about having an impact on the external world, which is a key part of being able to achieve goals. The broad, multidisciplinary interest in narrative as a mode of understanding that has emerged in recent decades has highlighted the ways in which the stories that we tell are structured around themes of agency, intentionality, purpose, and responsibility (Bruner, 1990; McAdams, 1993; McLeod, 1997). These perspectives offer a deeper appreciation of the meaning and significance of therapist/client talk about goals.

It may be helpful to think about therapy as comprising two contrasting forms of explanatory work. Scientifically informed causal analysis of a client's problems, leading to identification of strategies around what usefully can be done to bring about change, represent one dimension of explanatory work. The other explanatory dimension consists of exploring the purposefulness, intentionality, and agency of the client, leading to identification of goals. Within therapy, as within life in general, goal statements function as plausible explanatory accounts of human action: for instance, 'she changed her occupation *because* she wanted (goal) to be able to spend more time with her children'; 'she devoted time and energy in therapy to learning to be more assertive, *in order to* be able to make an important career shift'. These statements, which make perfect sense to most people, are examples of teleological reasoning—causation is attributed to an end-state. What is also obvious to most people is that such statements do not deny the existence or utility of a parallel explanatory account framed in cause-effect terms, for example 'her own childhood experience had taught her the importance of a mother spending time with her children', or 'developing a relationship of trust with her therapist was a necessary factor in becoming able to accept her own inner power'.

Some theories of therapy place a strong emphasis on the exploration and articulation of desires, wishes, and goals. Other theories tend to emphasize the analysis of causal sequences through which problems arise and are maintained. The existence of two contrasting dimensions of explanatory work suggests that, in practice, it may be valuable to ensure that *both* ways of thinking are given sufficient space within the process of therapy. It seems likely that effective therapists, within any school of practice, are able to facilitate a productive creative tension between these contrasting and complementary modes of understanding.

The experience of time

Western culture has generated a rich tradition of philosophical thought that seeks to develop ways of reconciling basic aspects of being human in the face of the massive social, technological, and environmental change that characterises our era in history. The writings of existential and phenomenological thinkers have functioned as a valuable resource for many people in contemporary societies, and particularly for psychotherapists and those looking for meaning in an increasingly fragmented world. The aim of phenomenology is to uncover and describe the essence of the experience of being human. One of the key aspects of this essence, described by Husserl, Heidegger, and other phenomenologists, is the sense of existing in time (Moran, 2000). What these philosophers are saying is that awareness of time is a bedrock of human experience. It is always there, whether or not we are consciously attending to it.

There have been two main ways in which awareness of time has been developed as a point of focus in psychotherapy. Clients talk about the past, in terms of what has gone wrong and how past events shape their present difficulties. Alternatively, clients are often encouraged, one way or another, to pay attention to present-moment experiencing, as a means of grounding themselves in authentic ways of relating to others, or to report on their lived experience of being anxious, or obsessive, or whatever. However, awareness of time also involves awareness of the future. In therapy, goals conversations represent a way of inviting the client to disclose their experience of future time.

Therapy goals can be fairly prosaic: for example, 'I want to be able to allow myself to feel good when someone says something nice to me'. Such a statement can open up a personal landscape for the future, as it can evoke other phenomenologically 'essential' aspects of human existence, such as choice and finitude/death. Exploring a statement such as 'allowing myself to feel good when someone says something nice to me' may lead to a personal confrontation with a realization that, to do this, I also need to decide that I am worthy of compliments in spite of my many imperfections, that I am not the utterly hopeless and unworthy person I have considered myself to be up to that point. Further exploration may readily introduce themes associated with finitude and death: for example, 'I do not want to die knowing that I have lived a life in which I have not allowed myself to receive love'.

The concept of 'possible selves' offers one way for eliciting existentially deeper meanings associated with therapeutic goals (Markus & Nurius, 1986; Whitty, 2002). Inviting reflection on *who* one might want to be, or be like, reaches beyond questions around what one might want to do (goals).

Goals talk can bring therapy closer to everyday life

Within psychology, one of the ways in which teleological explanations have been dealt with has been to define end-states as drives, needs, or motives (see Chapter 3, this volume). For instance, the goal of wanting to learn how to hunt might be explained as resulting from socialization or even from evolutionary pressures. This type of re-framing acknowledges the necessity of goals, but conceptualizes goals as ultimately arising from causal mechanisms. Sadly, however, if behaviours are merely understood in relation to what might have caused them in the past, we lose an important perspective on human behaviour that relates to our being able to undertake changes in our lives.

Conceptually, it is important in therapy to be aware that client talk about needs and motives is quite different from talk about goals. Conversations about goals in therapy refer to a complex landscape of action that breaks down into a shifting array of ongoing personal projects of greater or lesser degrees of significance for the client. What this means for therapy is that inviting clients to identify their goals for therapy represents an entry-point into a shared exploration of the way that they live their lives, in terms of the time and priorities allocated to different projects.

Theories of personality seek to make sense of the characteristics and development of individual identity and patterns of behaviour. Personality theory and research is highly relevant for applied fields of psychology, such as counselling and psychotherapy, because practitioners inevitably deal with individual differences between clients, and draw on personality theory to understand these differences. Historically, since the mid-twentieth century, the study of personality has been dominated by the concept of 'traits'—stable, recurring patterns of behaviour such as extraversion or neuroticism. Traits are essentially decontextualized entities—they represent patterns that are exhibited regardless of setting or culture. In addition, the concept of traits does not draw attention to human agency or choice. In recent years, there has been a sustained effort within the domain of personality psychology to find a means of making sense of why people behave differently (McAdams, 2013; McAdams & Pals, 2006). One of the approaches that has emerged as potentially valuable has been to understand individual differences in terms of the structure of personal projects being pursued by an individual (Little, 2014, 2015; Presseau et al., 2008; see Chapter 3, this volume). A personal project can encompass a wide range of possibilities, for example 'deciding on the best place to go on vacation next year', 'losing weight', and 'working to prevent climate change'. Research into personal projects analysis supports the value of this perspective as a means of enhancing self-awareness of individuals, as well for providing information that is useful for therapists and other practitioners (Egan, Scott-Lowery, De Serres Larose, Gallant, & Jaillet, 2016). When looked at as a whole, the structure of personal projects being pursued by an individual readily illustrates what is most important for the person (hierarchy of projects), areas of conflict between different projects, and evidence of change over the life course.

The language of goals

From a social constructionist perspective, human action, and the meaning that it has for individuals and groups, is mediated through language (Gergen, 1991, 2009a, 2009b). Historically, the words that we use and the ways that we talk with each other can be viewed as reflecting a complex cultural archaeology (Foucault, 1980) in which new meanings are built on previous forms of discourse, which themselves continue to resonate within these emergent ways of talking. Two main lines of research and inquiry have been influenced by this philosophical position. One area of focus has been how social realities and relationships are constructed within conversational interaction. This topic is addressed in the following section. The other area of focus has been to analyse the significance of word choice, in terms of the discursive traditions and positions that words, phrases, and images evoke.

The issue of word choice is of crucial importance when working with goals in therapy. There exist several different ways of referring to goals, each of which have subtly divergent meanings and implications for both clients and therapists.

In the following discussion, for reasons of space it will be assumed that clients and therapists are members of a shared culture and therefore likely to be influenced by the same set of cultural meanings. In practice, therapists tend to have been socialized into professional language communities that have their own distinctive ways of talking, and clients typically come from a much wider range of language contexts.

The term 'goal' is a metaphor. For many people, their first reaction to the term 'goal' will be in terms of images of soccer or other team sports. Etymological analysis of the linguistic origins of the term suggests that, from its earliest recorded usage in the fifteenth century, it referred to the winning move in a (now unknown) game. In drawing comparison between two domains of meaning (life and games), the metaphor highlights some aspects of a phenomenon while downplaying others. The term game can tend to invoke a sense of playfulness while downplaying seriousness. Not achieving a goal, in a game, merely means that the game goes on. Achieving a goal, in a game, means that the game re-starts. These attributes may not apply to the experience of life.

While these meanings are implied, in the background, when a therapist uses the term 'goal', they are rarely explicitly discussed. Perhaps closer to awareness, for some clients and therapists, is their exposure to 'goals', and similar terms such as 'objectives' and 'targets' as part of oppressive management-speak in the workplace, where goals are used to continuously assess personal performance success and failure. Others may draw on a more constructive meaning of 'goals', in the form of participation in sport or fitness training (my target is to run further or faster every day).

In understanding how metaphors function within language and cognition, it is helpful to refer to the work of Lakoff and Johnson (1999). In their view, all of the concepts that we use begin as embodied metaphors that draw on some aspect of our actual physical reality and experience. Some metaphors become conventional or 'dead' in the sense of not being immediately recognizable as metaphorical, whereas others are more readily identifiable as figures of speech.

In their analysis of the metaphoric conceptualization of time, Lakoff and Johnson (1999) suggest that we (English-language speakers) talk about time from the point of view of an observer at the present who is facing toward the future, with the past behind them. This set of meanings is reflected in the way in which some people talk about goals in terms of a *journey*. Within this metaphor, purposefulness or goal-directedness can be discussed in terms of places and destinations, modes of transport, companions on a journey, taking time out to rest, bends/forks in the road, and so on. In relation to psychotherapeutic work, many clients and therapists experience this set of meanings as helpful and facilitative.

Some clients have difficulty imagining a future for themselves at all, and can find the term 'goal' difficult to handle. Terms such as 'wished-for' or 'dream' draw attention to the existence of imagination: the person standing in the now cannot see the future, but instead needs to imagine it. A valuable strategy that is opened up by this way of talking is to imagine oneself in that place that exists in the future ('imagine you are at the end of your life, and a child asks what were your best memories'). The concept of 'hope', as in a future event that is hoped-for, represents another way of talking about a wish or dream. Goals talk that draws on terms such as 'possibilities' and 'preferred' options, has the effect of evoking multiple potential goals, and the notion of making choices between them.

Within this wide array of ways of talking about goals, there are many possibilities for therapists and clients to find ways of talking about goals that are meaningful for them. A valuable account of one therapist's development around these issues can be found in an autobiographical paper written by Florence Kaslow (2002). Kaslow initially trained in a process-oriented psychodynamic approach to therapy, in which explicit identification of goals did not play a part. Over the course of a career she acquired skills and training in family and couples work, narrative therapy, and business consultancy, all of which called for attention to the diverse goals of multiple clients in a family or group. Part of this learning involved an appreciation, when talking about goals, that 'language is not innocent' (Andersen, 1996)—the terminology that she used had a significant impact on clients. Where Kaslow (2002) ended up was a collaborative style of therapy and consulting that centred on the joint construction of an *action plan*. Clearly, other therapists working in different contexts will arrive at other ways of talking about goals, appropriate to their circumstances and their approach to therapy. An important implication for practice here is that even if the concept of 'goal' is serviceable as a means of describing a general process that occurs in therapy, many (or most) therapists and clients will not use that actual terminology in their conversations together.

Case example: Working with possible selves in counselling with young people

Tom was 15 years of age, and had lost his way at school. He had started to skip classes, and avoided completing homework. Worried about his progress, his mother persuaded him to make an appointment with the school counsellor. Following an initial exploratory meeting, the counsellor asked Tom if he would be interested in joining a 9-week 'school-to-work' group that was starting after the vacation. Tom agreed to give it a try. School-to-work comprised a small group of students, was highly participative and experiential, and was oriented around the idea of identifying possible selves (i.e. what do you want to do/be when you leave school?) and identifying a plan for how to become that person. A key activity involved finding images of adults doing things that were appealing to the young person, and then talking about the characteristics and attributes of people in these roles. Other helpful activities included making contact with adults in the community who represented 'possible future selves'; and constructing a timeline that connected up their present situation with their hoped-for future work role, and specified tasks, roadblocks, and decision-points on that journey. All this was extremely helpful for Tom, who was able to map out a direction in life that included both his ideal possible self (being a professional footballer) as well as other options. While being a highly goal-oriented intervention, the group leaders did not use words such as 'goals' or 'objectives', but instead created activities and exercises that concretized these concepts at an experiential level. Further information about this approach can be found in Oyserman, Terry, and Bybee (2002).

The co-construction of goals

An important development in twentieth-century philosophy was a movement in the direction of highlighting the relational nature of human experience: to be a person involves being in a relationship (Gergen, 2009a; Macmurray, 1961). Even solitary thinking and monologue can be viewed as multivoiced and dialogical, a performance carried out in relation to an imagined inter-locutor (Bakhtin, 1986). Within psychotherapy, a relational perspective has similarly been highly influential. A relational standpoint has enormous significance for working with goals in psychotherapy, because it acts as a reminder that the way in which a person describes and explores therapeutic goals will be powerfully shaped by the relational context within which such a conversation takes place.

The experience of having a specific personal goal is generally shaped by the experience of how others have related to one's goals in the past, as well as to expectations of how others will relate to one's goals in the future. A person typically experiences his or her personal goals as problematic when his or her goals are ridiculed, ignored, and shamed, or viewed as having the potential to lead to interpersonal conflict. Generally, a person's goals are treated as problematic if they do not suit another person; that is, if they do not fit in with another person's goals. If a person generally senses that others are interested and not disturbed by their dreams, hopes, or desires, then having personal goals is not a cause for concern. Thus, goals are generally experienced as problematic because of the way we expect them to relate to other people's goals (Mackrill, 2010). How goals are addressed relationally in therapy is therefore highly significant.

The most straightforward way that therapeutic goals are relationally co-constructed arises from the observation that many clients find it hard to articulate what they want from therapy. Often, once a client has told their story at the start of therapy, their therapist needs to work hard to clarify the goal, or even offer a tentative formulation, before a clear sense of what the client wants becomes apparent. Thus, even when the therapist is doing little more than reflective empathic listening, they are providing necessary support for the act of goal definition. It seems likely that, the more skilfully the therapist facilitates this process, the more accurate and detailed the emerging goal definition will be.

Many therapists use self-report forms to assist their clients in defining and sharing their goals for therapy (see Chapter 6, this volume). Some of these forms are framed in terms of problems and difficulties ('What do you want to work on in therapy?'), whereas others invite the client to think in terms of goals ('Where do you want to get to, by the end of therapy?'). Some forms have space to list only one or two problems/goals, whereas others provide space for 10 or more items. There are also a range of additional questions that may be included, such as the seriousness of the problem/goal, how long it has bothered the person, and how hopeful they are about resolving/achieving it through therapy. Generally, such self-report forms are regarded merely as ways of recording information. From a relational perspective, however, they may be viewed as rituals or moments of social interaction. Initially, the therapist needs to say something to the client about why they are being asked to complete the form. After the form is filled in, the therapist can react with genuine interest and curiosity, or may respond in a more detached manner. The form itself may convey an implicit message that 'you are a person with problems' or 'you are a person with hopes and dreams'. These are just some of the ways in which goals forms can initiate certain types of conversation and awareness, and close down other types. On the whole, goals forms have a business-like style that evokes a sensible, justifiable, rational response, rather than a response that may be confused, at the edge of awareness, or embarrassing to disclose.

Over and above any discussion that may be triggered by goals forms completed by the client, it is probable that at least some of the ongoing flow of conversation in therapy will touch on the topic of what the client hopes to gain from therapy. It seems likely that there are many different conversational strategies that therapists use during such conversations. In one study, Oddli, McLeod, Reichelt, and Rønnestad (2014) analysed strategies used by experienced therapists for establishing agreement around goals in early sessions of therapy. What they found was that the therapists in their sample only rarely used the word 'goal', instead exhibiting a wide range of ways of inviting reflection on what the client wanted from therapy, for example by encouraging them to think about the future, or look at barriers to change, and talking about expectations. What came across is that these therapists were clearly interested in what their clients hoped to gain from therapy, they were also highly aware of the complexity of personal goals, and wished to avoid any risk of being constrained by explicit goal agreements that were not sufficiently nuanced.

The examples of co-construction of goals discussed above refer to processes of joint action within the therapy room. A further means through which goals are co-constructed consists of cultural discourses and narratives that may influence the client, the therapist, or both. Goals that are discussed in therapy also depend on cultural understandings about what therapy is for. The ideas of professional therapists about appropriate goals for therapy are documented in published goals inventories. Although the Bern Inventory of Treatment Goals (Grosse Holtforth & Grawe, 2002) is more broadly based than the inventories developed by Braaten (1989) and McNair and Lorr (1964), none of these instruments include the goal of assistance in dealing with practical everyday problems—a key goal identified in interviews with low-income women in therapy by Pugach and Goodman (2015). The goals that are pursued in an individual case appear to depend as much on the therapist who is seen, and the clinic in which they work, as on the client's reason for attending therapy (Philips, 2009). The point here is that the institutional setting in which therapy is conducted, can convey subtle messages about what we talk about here, and what we do not.

An appreciation of the relational co-construction of therapy goals invites a more differentiated understanding of what happens during goals conversations in therapy sessions. For example, it makes it clear that the direction of causality is not just one way. The quality of the interaction between therapist and client may have an impact on the honesty with which a client reports his or her goals for therapy. However, there is also a process of reciprocal causality, in which the expression of goals feeds back into the therapeutic process. Client-therapist agreement around goals is generally considered to be a key aspect of the therapeutic alliance, and the process of completing and discussing a goals form may reinforce the confidence of both parties that such agreement does exist. This, in turn, helps to build a collaborative connection that enables goals to be talked about more openly. By contrast, lack of clarity around goals (i.e. avoidance of goals talk) may contribute to a weaker alliance that then in turn makes it harder to explore goals.

Case example: Isobel's battle with long-term illness

Isobel was 54 at the time of entering therapy. Diagnosed with multiple sclerosis (MS) nine years earlier, she felt depressed and defeated. Therapy was a last resort, and she had no idea about how it might help her, or what she might want to achieve through it. After three meetings, she was able to identify a couple of goals: 'to make a positive change in the way I feel about myself in relation to having MS', and 'to accept the reality of my illness, for example allowing members of the family to take care of me'. Isobel's therapist used an approach that emphasized collaboration and clarity around goals. Over time, as the client-therapist relationship deepened, and they became able to talk more honestly with each other, further goals emerged: 'becoming more assertive with unhelpful health professionals'; 'expressing anger in appropriate ways'; 'facing up to death and making plans for assisted suicide'. Progress in relation to early goals seemed to give Isobel the courage to formulate new goals that previously had been beyond meaningful consideration. In a research interview at the end of therapy, Isobel identified collaborative contracting and goal-setting as helpful aspects of the therapy she had received. Isobel's goal-setting developed during the course of her therapy and as an ongoing part of her therapy. Further discussion of how therapy goals changed in this case, and how the process of talking about goals made a tangible contribution to the process of therapy, can be found in McLeod (2013).

Ethical and value dilemmas

In therapy, the process of exploring the goals of a client is oriented toward learning about what that particular individual wants from life. However, the goals expressed by a client are not only personal strivings, but also reflect broader social and cultural ideas and values around what is considered important in life (MacIntyre, 1981). Taylor (1989) argues that human action is morally guided by stories of the 'good life': what people should do with their lives. We learn about the good life through a range of moral sources, in the form of stories available in religious texts, political agendas, movies, newspaper articles, and other sources. In societies that are dominated by strict religious teachings, there may exist a single good life narrative that specifies the purpose of life. By contrast, psychotherapy has developed in modern pluralistic societies where multiple stories of the good life sit alongside each other.

Therapy can be understood as a means of promoting a distinctive moral vision, reflected in a broadly humanistic ethos that values authentic relationships as opposed to material success (Christopher, 1996). As a result, the values and personal goals espoused by therapists may differ from those held by clients, thereby exacerbating the possibility of a values conflict. The goals of clients can be regarded as referring not only to practical issues around how to cope with relationship difficulties and stress, but also as a reflection of underlying moral dilemmas and choices. The values dimension of working with goals in therapy can therefore be hard to handle, because therapists are generally wary about exploring values issues. There is a fear of coming across as judgemental or persecutory to a client, or as using the therapeutic relationship to recruit the client to the moral position espoused by the therapist. Values differences between therapists and clients have been found to be associated with early dropout from treatment (Vervaeke, Vertommen, & Storms, 1997). So while exploration of client values associated with their therapeutic and personal goals is potentially facilitative, this is a topic that calls for a high level of therapist skill and sensitivity.

For some therapists, the moral vision that informs their work may be guided by a relational ethical stance that, following Levinas, places 'an emphasis on honouring the Other, *in all their otherness*' (Cooper, 2009, p. 121). This orientation to therapy involves a commitment to recognizing and affirming the ways in which that person is unique, active and reflective, and different from oneself, as a primary and fundamental activity within therapy (Sayre, 2005). One of the concrete ways in which this perspective can be expressed by therapists is to be curious about the client's goals for therapy, and respond to the client as an intentional and purposeful being. Another way of looking at this ethical perspective is to consider what it might mean, in moral terms, to *avoid* clarification of client goals.

Within the domain of professional ethics, working with client goals opens up issues around autonomy and informed consent. In relation to the ethical principle of individual autonomy, avoidance of clarification around client goals could be regarded as an ethical breach, as it would make it impossible to know whether the direction and focus of therapy was congruent with the client's views. That is, some kind of explicit checking-out of therapeutic goals is a necessary aspect of respect for client autonomy. The nature of autonomy is given particular prominence when the client is mandated to attend therapy because of a court order, where the goal of therapy has been specified by the court (e.g. to address issues around alcohol abuse or domestic violence) (Dwyer, 2012). Similar issues arise in other forms of third-party referral, such as a school student being referred to counselling by a teacher for the purpose of modifying disruptive behaviour.

When working with families, being aware of and reflecting on goals may become a way of drawing attention to significant ethical issues. Family members will typically have different goals not just for their family life, but also for what they want to achieve in therapy. For example, a teenager in a family may be hoping for more independence, whereas the parent seeks to restrict their independence. Parents may disagree vehemently about how to influence their children's behaviour, while each strives to find support for their view from the therapist. A young girl may fear physical and emotional abuse and long to be cared for and protected by a grandparent, a goal that she dare not voice in the presence of her parents, and that she fears telling a counsellor. A mother may strive to get her husband to stop drinking and aim to have her children support her in this endeavour. In cases such as these, goals are not just part of a way to manage therapy, they are also a window that offers access to key therapeutic issues in the case. In family therapy, disagreement about goals is to be expected, and exploring differences in goals is often part of the therapy process. If clear goal agreement was deemed to be a prerequisite for family therapy, many families would be deprived of help.

The practice of obtaining informed consent for participation in therapy comprises a specific aspect of the broader principle of autonomy. Informed consent usually focuses on issues that are common to all clients being seen at a particular service, such as confidentiality, fees, the type of therapy being offered, and appointment scheduling. Fisher and Oransky (2008) proposed that good ethical practice should also include consent around the goals of therapy. Clarification and agreement around goals may not be possible until two or three sessions into therapy (Pomerantz, 2005), with the implication that consent needs to be checked out at different points in time, rather than only at the start of the therapy (process consent). An important implication of this area of ethical practice is that it is essential to take particular care around clients who have difficulty in giving consent to therapeutic goals, either because they are not clear about their goals, or because they have a limited capacity to envisage such goals on account of age or cognitive processing difficulties. For example, during initial history-taking, a young client may mention that she experiences flashbacks to earlier experiences of sexual abuse, and also that she lacks confidence in social situations. The client may be keen to attend counselling, but remain vague around what she wants to achieve in therapy. It would be ethically problematic for a counsellor, in such a case, to initiate exploration of either of these topics in any depth, until a clear goals agreement was reached.

Case example: Joe's 'depression'

Joe was a 39-year-old Chinese American, whose grandparents escaped from communist oppression and established themselves in the USA. He was professionally successful, married with children. Although his employer persuaded him to see a therapist, Joe was not clear about how therapy might help him. On taking Joe's history, and observing him in the room, his therapist came to the conclusion that Joe was depressed. One goal for therapy, therefore, might be to overcome depression. Other people in Joe's life expressed different goals for him. His boss wanted Joe to be more productive. His children 'just want their Dad back, so we can have fun'. His traditionalist parents wanted Joe to be a devoted son who would attend to their needs. His wife wanted him to be a less devoted son, and more attentive husband. Somewhere in all of that, sat Joe's own wishes and hopes. In this case, clarification and identification of therapeutic goals were inextricably linked to ethical issues. For example, if Joe was depressed at a significant level of severity, was he emotionally and cognitively capable of expressing what he wanted from therapy? Was it morally appropriate for his therapist to define Joe's goals from an individualistic, American perspective, rather than from the more collectivist perspective of his family of origin? In the case of Joe, there were many directions that therapy might follow, depending on the goals that were agreed. However, to arrive at goal consensus, Joe and his therapist needed to find shared moral ground, through exploring the values positions that underpinned different goals. Further exploration of the moral and ethical dimensions of this case can be found in Tjeltveit (2006).

A further moral dimension of working with goals can be found in the 'human capabilities' approach developed by Martha Nussbaum and Amartya Sen. The concept of human capabilities has been highly influential in relation efforts to assert human rights and equality at a global level. Nussbaum (2011) proposes that there are certain core areas of human capability to which everyone has a right, such as being able to have good health, having opportunities for sexual satisfaction, being able to use imagination, and being able to have attachments and to love. Individual life projects and goals can be regarded as the expression of human rights in a particular person's everyday life. Human capability theory is therefore consistent with goal-informed therapy practice that aims to give clients permission to express and pursue their goals. This perspective may be useful in some therapy settings, in drawing attention to some of the ways in which goals conversations reflect a broader context of commitment to basic human rights.

The lived experience of goal-setting

The earlier sections of this chapter have explored various aspects of the process of working with client goals in therapy. A potentially valuable way to bring together the themes that have been discussed is to consider goal-exploration as a particularly complex type of lived experience. It is important, therefore, to ensure that research into goal-informed therapy takes account of this position. Qualitative research offers a systematic methodology for developing an understanding of the lived experience of persons in particular contexts, or who are facing particular life issues. There exists a growing qualitative research literature around the lived experience of goal-setting in such fields as nursing, occupational therapy, medicine, and organizational psychology (see, for example, Bateman & Barry, 2012; Brown, Bartholomew, & Naik, 2007; Doig, Fleming, Cornwell, & Kuipers, 2009; Lawler, Dowswell, Hearn, Forster, & Young, 1999; Schulman-Green, Naik, Bradley, Mccorkle, & Bogardus, 2006; Williams, Steven, & Sullivan, 2011). These studies have made a substantial contribution to an appreciation of the multiple processes that are associated with this kind of professional activity. The relative absence of qualitative research into working with goals in psychotherapy represents a crucial gap in the therapy evidence base.

Conclusions

The aim of the present chapter has been to examine conceptual and philosophical perspectives that may have the potential to take our understanding of goal-informed therapy to another level. What seems to be clear is that it is essential to acknowledge the complexity of the process of working with client goals, and find ways to incorporate essential epistemological, psychological, and ethical dimensions of this area of practice. Acknowledgement of complexity has important implications for counsellor and psychotherapist training. For example, it seems likely that, to make effective use of goals forms, trainees need help to make sense of the multiple levels of meaning and significance that such simple acts can have for the client and the client-therapist relationship. Acknowledgement of complexity also opens up many interesting and exciting possibilities around innovative practice. For example, it may be better for some clients to explore goals through narrative means, such as story-writing (Whitty, 2002) or visual means, such as timelines and post-it notes on whiteboards (Oyserman, Terry, & Bybee, 2002) rather than through form-filling. Other directions for innovation may build on theory and research in the psychology of personality (Little, 2014; Markus & Nurius, 1986). Finally, there are important and challenging issues around integrating moral and ethical awareness into goal-oriented therapy. This set of issues is of particular significance because if the process of talking about goals, and using that information to guide therapy, feels 'wrong' to a client, or even to be experienced as a violation, then he or she is likely to withdraw from meaningful participation.

Points for reflection

- Identify a change episode in your own life. In what ways are you able to explain why this change occurred, in terms of prior events and influences (i.e. a causal explanation)? In what ways are you able to explain what happened in terms of goals, purposes, and intentions (i.e. a teleological explanation)? What are the strengths and limitations of each type of explanation?

- Take a few minutes to make a list of the main life goals that are important for you at this time. Talk to someone else, a person you can trust, about these goals, for at least 30 minutes. The role of the other person is merely to listen, clarify that they have understood, and encourage you to talk. What differences were you aware of, between the individual list, and what emerged in conversation? What are the implications of what you have learned from this exercise, for the process of facilitating the effective co-construction of goals in therapy?

- Identify two (or more) personal life goals or projects that appear to be mutually incompatible. For example: 'I want to travel the world' and 'I want to get a secure job so I can buy my own home'. What are the values positions that underpin each of these goals? Is there an overarching source of value that might allow you to bridge these competing goals?

◆ What were the 'acceptable' or socially approved life goals in the family and community within which you grew up? In what ways do you continue to be motivated to accomplish these goals? What new goals have you developed for yourself? What were the life experiences that contributed to the emergence of these new personal goals? What are the implications for your approach as a therapist (or any other helping role) of your reflections on these processes of goal change?

Further reading

Bradley, E.H., Bogardus, S.T., Tinetti, M.E., & Inouye, S.K. (1999). Goal-setting in clinical medicine. *Social Science and Medicine, 49*, 267–78.

Although not a psychotherapy study, this paper provides a useful discussion of the ways in which goals are influenced by both patient and clinician values.

Mackrill, T. (2010). Goal consensus and collaboration in psychotherapy—an existential rationale. *Journal of Humanistic Psychology, 50*, 96–107.

Exploration of an existential perspective on working with goals in therapy.

Michalak, J., and Holtforth, M.G. (2006). Where do we go from here? The goal perspective in psychotherapy. *Clinical Psychology: Science and Practice, 13*, 346–65.

An invaluable review of how goals have been conceptualized and studied in psychotherapy research and practice.

Smith, R. (2015). Agency: A historical perspective. In C.W. Gruber, M.G. Clark, S.H. Klempe, & J. Valsiner (Eds.) *Constraints of Agency: Explorations of Theory in Everyday Life*. (Annals of Theoretical Psychology Volume 12). New York: Springer.

An introduction to the ways in which theological and philosophical ideas about goals have been shaped by social, cultural, and historical influences.

References

Andersen, T. (1996). Language is not innocent. In F.W. Kaslow, (Ed.) *Handbook of relational diagnosis and dysfunctional family patterns* (pp. 119–25), New York: Wiley.

Bakhtin, M.M. (1986). *Speech Genres and Other Late Essays*. Austin, TX: University of Texas Press.

Bateman, T.S., & Barry, B. (2012). Masters of the long haul: Pursuing long-term work goals. *Journal of Organizational Behavior, 33*, 984–1006.

Braaten, L.F. (1989). The self-development project list-90. A new instrument to measure positive life attainment. *Small Group Behavior, 20*, 3–23.

Brentano, F. (1973). *Psychology from an Empirical Standpoint*, ed. and trans. by L. L. McAlister. London: Routledge.

Brown, V.A., Bartholomew, L.K., & Naik, A.D. (2007). Management of chronic hypertension in older men: An exploration of patient goal-setting. *Patient Education and Counseling, 69*, 93–99.

Bruner, J.S. (1990) *Acts of Meaning*. Cambridge, MA: Harvard University Press.

Christopher, J. C. (1996). Counseling's inescapable moral visions. *Journal of Counseling and Development, 75,* 17–25.

Cooper, M. (2009). Welcoming the Other: Actualising the humanistic ethic at the core of counselling psychology practice. *Counselling Psychology Review, 24,* 119–29.

Doig, E., Fleming, J., Cornwell, P. L., & Kuipers, P. (2009). Qualitative exploration of a client-centered, goal- directed approach to community-based occupational therapy for adults with traumatic brain injury. *American Journal of Occupational Therapy, 63*(5), 559–68.

Dwyer, S.A. (2012). Informed consent in court-involved therapy. *Journal of Child Custody, 9,* 108–25.

Egan, M., Scott-Lowery, L., De Serres Larose, C., Gallant, L., & Jaillet, C. (2016). The use of Personal Projects Analysis to enhance occupational therapy goal identification. *Open Journal of Occupational Therapy, 4,* Article 4. Available at: http://dx.doi.org/10.15453/2168-6408.1186

Fisher, C.B., &. Oransky, M. (2008). Informed consent to psychotherapy: Protecting the dignity and respecting the autonomy of patients. *Journal of Clinical Psychology, 64,* 576–88.

Foucault, M. (C. Gordon, Ed.) (1980). *Power/knowledge: Selected interviews and other writings, 1972-1977.* New York: Pantheon Books.

Frankl, V. E. (1984). *Man's search for meaning.* New York: Washington Square Press.

Gergen, K.J. (1991) *The Saturated Self: Dilemmas of Identity in Modern Life.* New York: Basic.

Gergen, K.J. (2009a). *Relational Being: Beyond Self and Community.* New York: Oxford University Press.

Gergen, K.J. (2009b). *An Invitation to Social Construction,* 2nd edition. Thousand Oaks, CA: Sage.

Grosse Holtforth, M., & Grawe, K. (2002). Bern inventory of treatment goals: Part 1: Development and first application of a taxonomy of treatment goal themes. *Psychotherapy Research, 12,* 79–99.

Haynes, S.J., O'Brien, W.H., Kaholokula, J.K., & Witteman, C. (2012). Concepts of causality in psychopathology: applications in clinical assessment, clinical case formulation and functional analysis. *Journal of Unified Psychotherapy and Clinical Science, 1,* 87–103.

Heidegger, M. (2010) *Being and Time,* trans. by Joan Stambaugh, revised by Dennis J. Schmidt. Albany, NY: State University of New York Press. (Original work published 1927)

Kaslow, F.W. (2002). Shifting from treatment plans to action plans: solidifying the therapeutic alliance. *Journal of Contemporary Psychotherapy, 32,* 83–92.

Kierkegaard, S. (1843/1938). Journals. Vol. IV (A. Dru, Trans.). In J. Chamberlain & J. Rée (Eds.), *The Kierkegaard reader.* Oxford, UK: Blackwell.

Lakoff, G., & Johnson, M. (1999). *Philosophy in the flesh. The embodied mind and its challenge to Western thought.* New York: Basic Books.

Lawler, J., Dowswell, G., Hearn, J., Forster, A., & Young, J. (1999). Recovering from stroke: A qualitative investigation of the role of goal setting in late stroke recovery. *Journal of Advanced Nursing, 30,* 401–9.

Little, B.R. (2014). Well-doing: Personal projects and the quality of lives. *Theory and Research in Education, 12,* 329–46.

Little, B.R. (2015). The integrative challenge in personality science: Personal projects as units of analysis. *Journal of Research in Personality, 56,* 93–101.

Mackrill, T. (2010). Goal consensus and collaboration in psychotherapy—an existential rationale. *Journal of Humanistic Psychology, 50,* 96–107.

Maclntyre, A. (1981). *After Virtue: A Study in Moral Theory.* London: Duckworth.

Macmurray, J. (1961). *Persons in Relation.* London: Faber.

Markus, H., & Nurius, P. (1986). Possible selves. *American Psychologist, 41,* 954–69.

McAdams, D.P. (1993) *The Stories We Live By: Personal Myths and the Making of the Self.* New York: William Murrow.

McAdams, D.P. (2013). The psychological self as actor, agent, and author. *Perspectives on Psychological Science, 8,* 272–95.

McAdams, D.P., & Pals, J.L. (2006). A new Big Five: Fundamental principles for an integrative science of personality. *American Psychologist, 61,* 204–17.

McLeod, J. (1997). *Narrative and psychotherapy.* London: Sage.

McLeod, Julia. (2013). Transactional Analysis psychotherapy with a woman suffering from Multiple Sclerosis; a systematic case study. *Transactional Analysis Journal, 43,* 212–23.

McNair, D. M., & Lorr, M. (1964). Three kinds of psychotherapy goals. *Journal of Clinical Psychology, 20,* 390–3.

Moran, D. (2000). *An introduction to phenomenology.* London: Routledge.

Nussbaum, M. (2011). *Creating Capabilities: The Human Development Approach.* Cambridge, MA: Harvard University Press.

Oddli, H.W., McLeod, J., Reichelt, S., & Rønnestad, M.H. (2014). Strategies used by experienced therapists to explore client goals in early sessions of psychotherapy. *European Journal of Psychotherapy and Counselling, 16,* 245–66.

Oyserman, D., Terry, K., & Bybee, D. (2002). A possible selves intervention to enhance school involvement. *Journal of Adolescence, 25,* 313–26.

Philips, B. (2009). Comparing apples and oranges: How do patient characteristics and treatment goals vary between different forms of psychotherapy? *Psychology and Psychotherapy: Theory, Research and Practice, 82,* 323–36.

Pomerantz, A.M. (2005). Increasingly informed consent: discussing distinct aspects of psychotherapy at different points in time. *Ethics & Behavior, 15,* 351–360.

Presseau, J., Sniehotta, F.H., Francis, J.J., & Little, B.R. (2008). Personal projects analysis: Opportunities and implications for multiple goal assessment, theoretical integration, and behaviour change. *The European Health Psychologist, 10(2).* Available at: http://ehps.net/ehp/index.php/contents/article/view/ehp.v10.i2.p32/40

Pugach, M.R. & Goodman, L.A. (2015). Low-income women's experiences in outpatient psychotherapy: A qualitative descriptive analysis. *Counselling Psychology Quarterly, 28,* 403–26.

Sayre, G. (2005). Toward a therapy for the Other. *European Journal of Psychotherapy, Counselling and Health, 7,* 37–47.

Schulman-Green, D.J., Naik, A.D., Bradley, E.H., Mccorkle, R., & Bogardus, S.T. (2006). Goal setting as a shared decision making strategy among clinicians and their older patients. *Patient Education and Counseling, 63,* 145–51.

Taylor, C. (1989). *Sources of the Self.* Cambridge, MA: Harvard University Press.

Tjeltveit, A. (2006). To what ends? Psychotherapy goals and outcomes, the good life, and the principle of beneficence. *Psychotherapy: Theory, Research, Practice, Training, 43*, 186–200.

Vervaeke, G.A.C., Vertommen, H., & Storms, G. (1997). Client and therapist values in relation to drop-out. *Clinical Psychology and Psychotherapy, 4*, 1–6.

Whitty, M. (2002). Possible selves: Exploring the utility of a narrative approach. *Identity: An International Journal of Theory and Research, 2*(3), 213–30.

Williams, B., Steven, K., & Sullivan, F. M. (2011). Tacit and transitionary: an exploration of patients' and primary care health professionals' goals in relation to asthma. *Social Science & Medicine, 72*, 1359–66.

Chapter 3

The psychology of goals: A practice-friendly review

Mick Cooper

The overarching goal of this chapter is to review psychological evidence and theory on goals and goal processes, and to draw out implications for clinical practice. More specifically, drawing on the research, the goals of this chapter are to critically discuss:

- the relationship between goals and affect;
- key dimensions along which goals can vary;
- the nature of goal processes, such as planning and disengaging from goals;
- a hierarchical framework for understanding the relationship between goals;
- the relationship between goals and the social context;
- the implications of these analyses for therapeutic practice.

'Since the 1980s', write Grouzet *et al.* (2005, p. 800), 'psychological research on goals has experienced a real renaissance'. This has been in a number of areas: for instance, the impact of goal-setting on task performance (e.g. Locke & Latham, 2002), the relationship between goals and wellbeing (e.g. Elliot & Church, 2002), and the neuropsychology of goals (e.g. Reeve & Lee, 2012). For Cooper and Joseph (2016), such psychological research can form an importance basis for therapeutic practice. Like the roots of a tree, they argue, psychological knowledge can, 'provide nourishment and stimulation for growth … fuelling new ideas and practices that can be tested out, researched, and refined' (pp. 12–13). Moreover, they suggest that it can, 'provide a "grounding" for psychotherapeutic practice: ensuring that it is embedded in valid and defensible models of human functioning and change' (p. 13).

Clearly, psychological evidence cannot be considered the only important source on which to base clinical practice, nor an infallible one. For instance, psychological knowledge is often based on settings and samples that are unrepresentative of the clinical context, and generally neglects the domain of subjective lived-experiences. However, given that it may provide some important insights into clinical work, the aim of this chapter is to review the psychological research and theory on goals and goal processes, and to explore its relevance for clinical practice. The approach taken here is of a 'practice-friendly' review (Mcleod, 2012), where there is a particular emphasis on establishing guidance for therapeutic work.

Unfortunately, the psychological research and theory focuses mainly on adults rather than children and young people, and therefore discussion of the latter will be limited. However, wherever possible, research, theory, and implications for work with children and young people also will be considered.

Goals, wellbeing, and affect

Why might goals be important to the work that therapists do? One answer to this question, as suggested by a growing body of psychological evidence, is that it is because goals and goal-related processes are fundamental to how positive or negative people feel. More specifically, the evidence suggests five particular ways in which people's feelings of positive or negative affect tend to be related to their goals (see, Wiese, 2007).

First, as meaning-centred therapists have argued (e.g. Frankl, 1984), the *awareness* that one has goals and purposes, and the belief that they are meaningful and important, is associated with wellbeing (Little, Salmela-Aro, & Phillips, 2007). Indeed, Emmons and Diener (1986) found that 'positive affect is just as strongly related to having important goals as it is to the attainment of these goals' (p. 315). Consistent with this, research has demonstrated abundant links between a sense of meaning and purpose in life and other indicators of wellbeing (see Steger, 2013, for a comprehensive review). People with lower levels of purpose in life, for instance, have greater levels of psychological distress, more substance-related problems, and more disruptive behaviour. They also have lower levels of life satisfaction, self-esteem, positive affect, and physical functioning (King & Hicks, 2013; Park, Park, & Peterson, 2010; Steger, 2013; Vos, 2016).

Second, research indicates that people tend to experience positive affect when they feel that their goals are *attainable*. That is, even without achieving or progressing towards their goals, people feel better if they believe that they will be successful in achieving important goals (Emmons, 1986); and that they have control, support, and opportunities to work towards their accomplishment (Brunstein, 1993).

Third, research indicates that *progress* towards goals (i.e. the subjective perception of moving towards them, as opposed to their actual attainment, Wiese, 2007) also tends to lead to enhance feelings of wellbeing and positive affect

(Brunstein, 1993; Wiese, 2007). In the most comprehensive meta-analysis to date, Koestner *et al.* (2002) found that 'Participants reported significantly more positive affect and less negative affect over time when they had made greater goal progress' (p. 233).

Fourth, positive affect may be related to the *rate* of progress towards goals, as well as to progress, itself. Here, Carver and Scheier (1990; 2012) have hypothesized that people will experience positive affect when they are moving towards their goals at a rate higher than standard, negative affect when the rate is lower than standard, and no affect when they are progressing at a standard rate. This means, for example, that I could be progressing towards a goal but still experiencing frustration, because my rate of progress is much slower than I had expected. However, to date, evidence in support of this hypothesis is 'sparse' (Wiese, 2007, p. 311).

Finally, research indicates that people tend to feel good when they *achieve* their goals (Sheldon & Elliot, 1999; Wiese, 2007). Emmons and Diener (1986), for instance, found a large positive correlation of .46 between the attainment of goals and positive affect; while Sheldon and Elliot (1999) found a moderate positive correlation of .34. Goal achievement is likely to feel good both because of the affect generated by a successful goal process, but also because of the affect generated by the goal-object, itself. For instance, if I achieve my goal of establishing a close, intimate relationship, I have both the satisfaction of reaching the objective that I set for myself, but also the pleasure of experiencing a deep, connected relatedness.

Although research has tended to focus on the relationship between goals and relatively global positive or negative affect, if 'affect serves as feedback indicating that either progress towards goals is being made or that important goals have been attained' (Emmons & Diener, 1986, p. 311), then it may be possible to specify more clearly what emotions arise in relation to particular goal processes. For instance, as Ryan and Deci (2008) state, anger or sadness could be associated with having our goal thwarted. In this respect, Table 3.1 lists hypotheses of the particular kinds of positive and negative affect that may arise in relation to the presence or absence of particular goal processes.

In summary, then, people tend to experience positive affect when they are oriented towards goals, see them as attainable, feel that they are progressing towards them (and, ideally, at a faster-than-expected rate), and achieve them. These processes can be referred to as the *actualization* of goals.

However, what the research also shows is that the affect invoked by these processes is also dependent on the type of goal being actualized, and it is to these moderators that we now turn.

Table 3.1 Emotions hypothesized to arise in the presence or absence of goal processes

	Presence	**Absence**
Awareness of goals	Meaning, purpose, sense of direction, orientation, order	Meaninglessness, disorientation, chaos, directionlessness, despair
Perceived attainability of goals	Hope, optimism, control, order, excitement, expectation	Hopelessness, futility, fear, anger, shame, sadness
Progress/velocity towards goals	Hope, accomplishment, excitement, self-belief, expectation, control, flow	Frustration, failure, despair, disillusionment, lack of self-belief, anger
Achievement of goals	Satisfaction, accomplishment, fulfilment; experiencing of the desired state, per se (e.g. relaxation, physical pleasure)	Dissatisfaction, failure, sadness, loss, frustration, envy, anger

Goal types

Within the adult psychological literature, several different taxonomies of goals have been proposed. For instance, Winell (1987) proposed six domains: career, family, leisure, social-community, personal growth, and materials; while Ford and Nichols (1987) detailed a comprehensive taxonomy of within-person goals (affective, cognitive, and subjective organization), and person-environment goals (self-assertive social relationship, integrative social relationships, and task) (cited in Austin & Vancouver, 1996). Within the therapeutic field, Holtforth and Grawe (2002) drew on data from approximately 300 adult outpatients to develop a taxonomy of clients' goals. This identified 23 types of goals, categorized into five main categories: interpersonal goals, coping with specific problems and symptoms, personal growth, wellbeing and functioning, and existential issues. Berking *et al.* (2005) found that adults in therapy were most likely to attain wellbeing goals, followed by interpersonal goals and personal growth goals, with existential goals least likely to be attained. Drawing on this taxonomy, Rupani *et al.* (2014) identified four categories of goals for young people in therapy—specific issues, personal growth, emotional issues, interpersonal issues—but did not find significant differences in goal attainment through therapy. Jacob *et al.* (2016), in a separate study of the goals of children and young people in therapy, also identified specific difficulties and personal growth goals, along with independence goals. Parents' and carers' goals for their children differed somewhat, with a greater emphasis on managing specific difficulties, parent-specified goals, and improving self or life.

Rather than proposing taxonomies, however, most researchers have tended to focus on the specific (albeit interrelated) dimensions across which goals might vary. Here, many different dimensions have been proposed. In his Personal Project Analysis, for instance, Little (1983) identified 27 different goal dimensions, including levels of 'visibility', 'challenge', and 'control'. Austin and Vancouver (1996), in their comprehensive review of the empirical and theoretical literature, suggest six main dimensions: (a) importance-commitment, (b) difficulty-level, (c) specificity-representation, (d) temporal range, (e) level of consciousness, and (f) connectedness-complexity.

Building on these frameworks, the following sections review eight key goal dimensions that may be of particular relevance to therapeutic practice. With the first four dimensions, there is clear evidence that these moderate the relationship between goal actualization and wellbeing. With the subsequent dimensions, the moderating effect is either hypothetical, or else inferred from evidence that the dimension moderates the degree of goal attainment (but not wellbeing, per se).

Importance

At a most basic level, goals can vary in their importance to a person. Some of my goals, for instance, are very important to me: like contributing towards a socially just society. Others are less important (albeit still goals): for instance, unpacking the boxes that have been sitting in my office for the past two years. The importance of goals to a person is closely connected to a range of other dimensions, such as the attractiveness, relevance, and accessibility of their goals (Austin & Vancouver, 1996). Also very closely connected, is a person's commitment to a particular goal. Here, research demonstrates that goal commitment mediates the relationship between goal-attainment and subjective wellbeing (Brunstein, 1993). That is, as might be expected, the more that a person is committed to achieving a particular goal, the better they feel when they perceive it as being attainable. However, the 'flip-side' of this is that, the more a person is committed to a particular goal, the worse they feel if that goal does not seem to be attainable. Hence, the more important goals are to people, the more their affective responses are likely to be heightened—in both positive and negative directions.

Important goals can also be considered similar to *core projects*: 'those that are more resistant to change, most extensively connected with other projects, and intrinsically valued by the person as pursuits without which the meaning of one's life would become compromised' (Little, 2007, p. 43). However, while the 'core-ness' of goals is likely to remain relatively stable over time, their importance may vary quite markedly. For instance, generally in my life, it is not a core project of mine to win at Trivial Pursuit (a quiz-based board game). However, in the midst of a challenge with friends or family, it can take on the utmost importance. Hence, there can be a discrepancy between core goals and goals that are experienced as important at particular moments in time. The potentially negative consequences of this—in the form of *rogue goals*—will be explored later on in the chapter.

Challenge

Some goals, like beating my nine-year-old son at Trivial Pursuit, are relatively easy to achieve. Other goals, like beating my wife at this game, are much more difficult. Goal challenge, or difficulty, can be defined as the 'level of knowledge and skill that is required to achieve a goal' (Sheeran & Webb, 2012, p. 178). Here, there is some evidence that goal difficulty mediates the relationship between goal progress and wellbeing, with people experiencing more positive affect when progressing towards more difficult goals (Wiese, 2007). That is, for example, if I start to beat my son at Trivial Pursuit, I do not feel a great deal of positive affect, because it is fairly expected. But starting to win against my wife generates some very noticeable positive feelings like satisfaction and glee.

Related to this, one of the strongest and most consistent findings in the goal-setting literature is that people tend to show greater progress when they act towards more difficult goals compared with easier ones (Locke & Latham, 2002; Wiese, 2007). For instance, if I set myself the goal of losing eight pounds in a month, I am likely to lose more weight than if I set myself the goal of losing one pound. And, to the extent that greater goal progress is associated with greater positive affect, then more challenging goals should lead to more positive feelings.

However, this is likely to be moderated by the degree to which a goal is realistic: a dimension closely related to levels of challenge. Although evidence is mixed (Sheeran & Webb, 2012), a highly challenging goal may be highly unrealistic, and therefore lead to greater feelings of negative affect because there is less goal progress or attainment. For instance, while I do feel better if I beat my wife at Trivial Pursuit compared with my son; in reality, I am less likely to experience positive affect when I play against my partner. And this is for the simple reason that the goal of beating her is less likely to be achieved: it is less realistic. Hence, the most *salutogenic* (i.e. facilitative of wellbeing) goals may be those that are challenging, but also realistic to achieve.

Approach vs. avoidance

In recent years, Elliot and colleagues (Elliot & Friedman, 2007) have argued that a fundamental distinction can be drawn between *approach*, and *avoidance*, goals. 'Approach goals are focused on a positive, desirable outcome or state and regulation entails trying to move toward or maintain the outcome or state' (Elliot & Church, 2002, p. 244). An example of this might be, 'having more friends'. By contrast, 'avoidance goals are focused on a negative, undesirable outcome or state and regulation entails trying to move or stay away from the outcome or state' (Elliot & Church, 2002, p. 244). An example of this might be, 'not being lonely'. Approach goals involve a 'promotion focus' (Higgins, 1997) and a sensitivity to gains, in which the person is trying to reduce the discrepancy between their current state and a desired one. By contrast, avoidance goals involve a 'prevention focus' and a sensitivity to losses, in which the person is trying to maximize the discrepancy between their current state and a feared one. Elliot and colleagues (Elliot & Church, 2002) argue that such a distinction is of so much importance that it can be considered the highest order division between goals. Indeed, as with 'regulatory focus theory' (Higgins, 1997), they argue that people can be characterized according to whether they have a basic approach/promotion orientation, or a basic avoidance/prevention one.

This distinction between approach and avoidance goals is of particular importance to a therapeutic context because 'Recent research has linked avoidance goal regulation to a host of negative processes and outcomes' (Elliot & Church, 2002, p. 244). For instance, Elliot and Sheldon (1997) found that a focus on avoidance, rather than approach, goals was associated with lower subjective wellbeing, adjustment, and experience. More specifically, within the therapeutic context, Elliot and Church (2002) showed that clients who adopted more avoidance goals evidenced smaller increases in wellbeing from the start to the end of therapy, experienced less goal progress, and were less satisfied with the work. Similarly, Wollburg and Braukhaus (2010) found that clients with more avoidance goals showed less reductions in depression symptomatology.

There may be a number of reasons for the negative effects of avoidance goals. First, in contrast to approach goals, there is no clear end state that can be achieved. A person striving for more friends, for instance, can know when they have achieved this goal and move on; but a person trying to avoid loneliness can never fully know if they have achieved their objective, as there is always the possibility that the feared state will return. Second, closely linked to this, we are less likely to be successful in achieving avoidance goals because the warded off state, in most instances, simply cannot be eradicated. I may try and avoid failure, for instance, but it is inevitable that this will sometimes happen. Third, the means towards avoiding something is often less clear than the means towards approaching something. How do I avoid loneliness, for instance, when there are so many different ways in which it might be evoked? It is like trying to hold back the tide. By contrast, if I am trying to achieve something, I can create specific plans for myself (see 'Implementation intentions', this chapter). Moreover, as a fifth point, as I start to actualize approach goal plans, my sense of self-efficacy may increase, hence enhancing my capacity to achieve my goals. By contrast, successful avoidance is unlikely to leave me with a sense of achievement. Indeed, it may leave me with such negative feelings as cowardliness or being pathetic. Sixth, as Kahneman (2011) discusses, trying to avoid something is inherently problematic because it requires us to call to mind the thing we want to avoid, hence making it more salient. To try and avoid failure, for instance, I need to think about the ways in which I have failed, which reminds me of all the failings in my life. By contrast, thinking about positive approach goals is likely to evoke feelings of hope and optimism. Finally, research suggests that attempting to avoid negative goals may be more likely to generate acute, variable, and chaotic feelings, in contrast to the smoother process of approaching a desired state (Fujita & MacGregor, 2012).

Intrinsic vs. extrinsic

Another dimension of goals that has been widely discussed, and researched, in recent years is the degree to which the goal is *intrinsic*, or *extrinsic*, to the person. Intrinsic, or *self-concordant* goals (Sheldon & Elliot, 1999; Sheldon & Houser-Marko, 2001), are 'those that are likely to satisfy basic and inherent psychological needs' (Kasser & Ryan, 1996, p. 280), such as the need for relatedness and autonomy (Ryan & Deci, 2000). By contrast, *extrinsic* goals are those that 'primarily entail obtaining contingent external approval and rewards' (Kasser & Ryan, 1996, p. 280): for instance, the desire for wealth, appearance, and fame. This links closely to person-centred theory (Rogers, 1959) and its distinction between organismic needs and needs that are based on the desire for positive self- and other-regard. Research suggests that the intrinsic-extrinsic dimension is a critical moderator of the relationship between goal actualization and wellbeing, because it is only the actualization of intrinsic goals that leads to positive outcomes (Sheldon & Kasser, 1998). More specifically, while the pursuit of intrinsic goals is associated with higher levels of psychological wellbeing, greater satisfaction, and greater achievement of goals; the pursuit of extrinsic goals is associated with lower wellbeing, lower vitality, and more anxiety, depression, and physical symptoms (Kasser & Ryan, 1993, 1996, 2001; Koestner *et al.*, 2002; Sheldon & Elliot, 1999; Sheldon & Kasser, 1998).

This dimension bears many similarities to the distinction that has been made between *learning* (or *mastery) goals* and *performance goals* (Dweck & Leggett, 1988; Elliott & Dweck, 1988; Moskowitz & Grant, 2009b; Murayama, Elliot, & Friedman, 2012). Learning goals, like intrinsic goals, have an end in themselves: for instance, to acquire new knowledge, skills, and competencies. By contrast, performance goals, like extrinsic goals, are focused on achieving outcomes as a means of displaying competence to others: oriented towards external benchmarks and rewards, rather than being ends in themselves. As with the intrinsic-extrinsic dimension, there is evidence that learning goals tend to be more beneficial to the person than performance goals. For instance, performance goals are more likely to lead to feelings of helplessness after a failure, while learning goals facilitate persistence and mastery-oriented behaviours (Moskowitz & Grant, 2009b). To some extent, the intrinsic and extrinsic dimension also maps on to a distinction between 'process focus' and 'outcome focus', respectively, in goal-directed activity (Freund, Hennecke, & Mustafic, 2012).

Specificity

Goals can be specific and precise, or they can be vague and amorphous. An example of the former might be: 'To go the gym at least three times a week'. An example of the latter might be, 'To be fitter'. This dimension is closely related to the degree with which a goal is concrete, as opposed to abstract. Here, 'Concrete goals detail specific, tangible rewards achieved by particular behaviours in response to particular contexts. Abstract goals, in contrast, reflect more global, general aims that transcend specific situations and apply to multiple contexts' (Fujita & MacGregor, 2012, p. 86). The specificity of a goal is also closely associated to its simplicity, as opposed to its complexity. A complex goal, such as 'Getting fitter', is linked to a wide range of other goals and behaviours. It can be achieved through multiple pathways (see discussion of equifinality, later). By contrast, a simple goal, such as 'Going to the gym three times a week', is relatively distinct, and can be achieved through only a small number of means.

Generally, research shows that people perform better (i.e. make more progress towards the specified goal) when they aim for specific and simple goals, as opposed to goals that are vague and complex (Locke & Latham, 2002; Sheeran & Webb, 2012). However, in terms of wellbeing, this may be counterbalanced by a person's most important goals being relatively abstract: for instance, 'feeling that I am a lovable person'. Hence, while people may make progress when the goal is well-specified, if it is not that important to the person, then it may be less likely to evoke positive feelings of wellbeing.

Temporal extension

A closely related dimension of goals is their temporal extension: the degree to which they are long-term, distal 'life goals' (Pohlmann, 2001), as opposed to short-term, proximal objectives. This temporal extension can be defined in terms of how far in the future the goal object is, as well as the amount of time needed to know whether success or failure has been achieved (Fujita &

MacGregor, 2012). For instance, winning against my son at Trivial Pursuit is a proximal objective, because I know very shortly after we have started whether I have been successful or not. By contrast, my goal of helping to create a more socially just world is much more distal because it may take many years before I know if I have been successful or not—if ever.

Within the therapeutic field, we can make a specific distinction between 'life goals' (what the person wants to achieve, generally, in life), and the more proximal 'therapeutic goals' (what the person wants to achieve, specifically, in therapy) (Hanley, Sefi, & Ersahin, 2015; Mackrill, 2011). This distinction may be important as a means of helping to ensure that clients' goals are tailored to, and realistic within, the therapeutic context.

As with specific goals, research tends to suggest that the setting of more proximal goals generates more success than the setting of distal goals (Locke & Latham, 2002). However, as with specificity, the impact of temporal extension on wellbeing may be counterbalanced a person's most important goals being distal rather than proximal. My distal goal of helping to create a more just world, for instance, is much more important to me than my proximal goal of beating my son at Trivial Pursuit. Hence, even though the latter may be easier to achieve, the attainment of the former would be a far more significant source of positive affect.

Consciousness

'In many everyday cases', writes Chun *et al.* (2011), 'people's choices are guided by volitional goals of which they are acutely aware' (p. 1124). However, one of the most influential developments in the contemporary goals literature is the recognition that people's choices and behaviours can be influenced by unconscious, implicit goals (e.g. Marien, Custers, Hassin, & Aarts, 2012). Indeed, it has been argued that this may be the norm, rather than the exception (Austin & Vancouver, 1996; Moskowitz & Grant, 2009a). An example of this, within a therapeutic context, is given by Cooper and McLeod (2011, pp. 64-5):

> Jennifer was a client who had been sexually abused in childhood, and wished to use therapy to help her to come to terms with what had happened, and to get rid of painful and frightening memories of what had happened. Over the course of several months, however, Jennifer seemed to find it hard to commit herself to therapy. Although she said that she liked her therapist, and was satisfied with the way that the therapist was working with her problems, she still missed several sessions, and on occasion could be quite sarcastic towards her, or remain silent and withdrawn for lengthy periods. At the same time, the therapist had a strong sense that it was essential that she should remain consistently accepting and caring in her responses to Jennifer, no matter what the provocation. Eventually, the therapist invited Jennifer to consider the possibility that some 'testing out' might be taking place, and if it was,

then what it might mean. What emerged from this discussion was an appreciation on both sides that Jennifer wanted a relationship in which she could feel unequivocally valued and 'special', and was trying to find out whether her therapist was someone who could provide this. Up until that conversation, the idea that 'finding a relationship in which I can feel valued and special' had not been a goal that Jennifer would have been capable of putting into words.

In support of such unconscious goal processes, Bargh and colleagues (e.g. Bargh & Ferguson, 2000) have demonstrated across numerous studies that goals can determine behaviours without people being consciously aware of them. For example, in a classic experiment, Bargh *et al.* (2001) first 'primed' some participants by asking them to undertake a sentence completion task that contained cooperation-related terms, such as 'helpful' and 'fair'. Subsequently, these participants behaved more cooperatively on a resource allocation 'game' than participants who had not had this priming. Crucially, however, these participants were not aware of any link between the two activities. In other words, they were acting towards the goal of being cooperative, but had no awareness of what this goal was, or that they had been directed towards it by the priming task.

In their work, Bargh and colleagues have also suggested that goals may be pursued so many times that they become *chronic*: that is, in a state of heightened accessibility across situations and time (Bargh, 1990). Furthermore, despite the unconscious status of these goals and the automaticity of behaviour towards them, research shows that unconscious goal pursuit can have many of the complex and adaptive features of conscious goal pursuit. For instance, people acting towards unconscious goals can display goal-related behaviour in novel settings; overcome obstacles; and use monitoring, feedback, and 'goal-shielding' processes (i.e. protecting the goal-related activity from distracting thoughts) to achieve their objectives (Aarts & Custers, 2012). We can see this in the example of Jennifer, discussed above, who employs such complex mechanisms as sarcasm and lengthy silences to achieve her goal of knowing another deeply cares for her.

In terms of how unconscious goal pursuit may take place, Aarts and Custers (2012) suggest that it is through the activation of positive, internal reward stimuli. That is, the representation of a particular outcome evokes positive feelings, such that we act towards that outcome without necessarily being aware of what it is. For instance, I might post videos of cats doing funny things on Facebook because it invokes in me a feeling of positive reward as I imagine all the people 'liking' me for it. However, I may never be conscious of those evoked positive feelings, or that rationale. Indeed, at a conscious level, I may believe that I am posting these for a very different reason: for instance, just to help everyone else have a happier day.

This links to the distinction made by McClelland *et al.* (1989) between *implicit* motives and *self-attributed* (or *explicit*) motives (as well as distinctions between 'latent' and 'manifest' goals, Murayama *et al.*, 2012). Here, McClelland *et al.* distinguish between those fundamental needs that arise early in a person's development, and the subsequent, conscious motives that a person attributes to themselves regarding what it is that they want. Crucially, McClelland *et al.* have argued that implicit motives (as assessed by such projective tests as the Thematic Apperception Test), and self-attributed motives (as assessed by self-report surveys) are independent. In fact, subsequent meta-analyses have shown some degree of association, but it is small (a correlation of .088, Spangler, 1992). In other words, research tends to support the hypothesis that the goals we consciously believe we have may be very different from those that are actually driving our behaviour. Furthermore, research suggests that it is the implicit motives, rather than the self-identified ones, that are most predictive of real-world behaviour. This is particularly the case where the behaviour is intrinsically rewarding. By contrast, when social incentives (such as external rewards) are present, self-identified motives may be more predictive of behaviour (Spangler, 1992).

However, evidence also exists that people vary quite considerably in the degree to which their goals are unconscious. Thrash *et al.* (2012) describe this as *motive congruence*: the degree of concordance between implicit and explicit motives. Drawing on the evidence, they suggest that motive congruence is higher in individuals who are more self-determining (i.e. regulating in accordance with their true, intrinsic motives), and whose early environment supported the development of self-determination by meeting their basic needs for autonomy and relatedness. They also suggest that individuals who are higher in motive congruence are more sensitive to their bodily states, less monitoring of other's expectations, and more concerned with self-consistency. Thrash *et al.* also cite research that lower levels of motive congruence are associated with lower levels of affective wellbeing over time.

Meta-level

A final dimension of goals—less explored in the psychological field, but of potential importance to therapy—is the *meta-level* of the goal. Most goals are of a *basic* type, in that the goal-object is a particular state or object. For instance, 'I want to go for a run'. However, it is also possible that the goal-object is a goal, or a goal-related process, itself. Examples of this might be the avoidance goal 'I don't want to have un-finished goals in my life' or the approach goal 'I must succeed in achieving my goals'. Note, to some extent, all goals related to the desire for competence can be seen, to some extent, as meta-level goals.

The concept of meta-goals may be particularly relevant to dysfunctional clinical processes because they introduce the possibility of vicious (as well as virtuous) cycles between goals. For instance, supposing that I have a meta-goal that I should not fail on any of my goals. Then, if I do fail (if, for instance, I don't go out for a run), then not only do I feel bad about that, but I also feel bad at the meta-goal level (I have failed at warding off failure). This, then, can spark off a vicious downward spiral of feeling that I have failed. That is, I experience failure because I have failed at my meta-goal, which intensifies my feeling of failure, *ad nauseam*. Compare this with the person whose meta-goal is to accept themselves whether they fail or succeed. Here, the person may still experience a sense of failure for not going for a run, but the process ends here.

Extending this discussion further, to the extent that affect is considered to be the result of goal-related processes (as discussed earlier), it could be argued that all emotion-related goals are essentially meta-goals. That is, if feeling happier is the result of progressing towards one's goals, then a goal of 'feeling happier' is essentially a goal about a goal-related process. This, again, raises the possibility for vicious and virtuous cycles. For instance, if a client's goal is that 'I don't want to feel unhappy', then a momentary experience of unhappiness may trigger a vicious downward spiral, in which their feelings of unhappiness evoke feelings of failure and unhappiness (for failing at their goal), which then evokes more feelings of distress. Concomitantly, however, the same person may experience a virtuous cycle at moments of joy, when a sense that they are achieving a goal of being happy may lead to feelings of satisfaction and success, which may then lead to more positive feelings of achievement.

Vicious and virtuous cycles may also arise between goals and emotions because, as the research demonstrates, negative affect may impede an individual's ability to follow through on their goals, while positive affect seems to facilitate goal-striving (Gollwitzer & Oettingen, 2012). This might be because negative feelings lower the person's sense of self-confidence, distract them, or reduce their levels of motivation or energy. The result, however, is that they are then less able to actualize their goal, hence enhancing the negative affect, which then impedes their abilities, *ad nauseam*. An example of this might be a student who is struggling to complete their assignment, who then feels bad about it, and who is then less able to focus on their work.

Goal processes

Within the psychological literature, there is also a body of research on how people go about actualizing their goals (see Gollwitzer & Oettingen, 2012). Some of this research focuses on the particular stages, or phases, that people go through in the goal pursuit process. These models tend to distinguish between a wanting phase, intentions, and actual behaviours. This is important as we can want things without intending them to happen; although intention does predict behaviour, it is not identical (e.g. Ajzen, 1991). Austin and Vancouver (1996) suggest four goal processes: establishing, planning, striving, and revising; while Little (1983) suggests a similar set: inception, planning, action, and termination. Somewhat more nuanced are the four action phases of the *Rubicon model* (Gollwitzer, 1990; Heckhausen & Gollwitzer, 1987). Here, the first phase is the *predecisional phase*, in which the person considers the desirability and feasibility of various wishes and wants. This culminates in a goal intention: that is, 'I intend to do X to attain Y'. This is where the person may 'cross the Rubicon' as the goal pursuit begins, at which point they can either succeed or fail. This is followed by the *preactional* phase, in which the individual arranges how to realize the goal. The third phase is the *action* phase, in which the planned behaviour is initiated and maintained. Finally, there is the *postactional* phase, in which the outcomes are evaluated against the goals and, if necessary, the cycle may be recommenced.

Mental contrasting

At the predecisional and preactional phases of goal-directed activity, research has focused on the process and value of *mental contrasting* (Oettingen & Stephens, 2009). This is a cognitive process in which the individual first imagines a desired future (e.g. 'Having a job in which I can express my creativity'), *and* then reflects on their current negative reality that stands in the way of that (e.g. 'There is no opportunity for creativity in my current role'). Within the 'theory of fantasy realization', mental contrasting can be contrasted with *indulging*, in which the person solely fantasizes about the positive future; and *dwelling*, in which the person merely ruminates on the negative reality. Mental contrasting has been shown to lead to greater goal commitment and goal-directed behaviour; and it is thought to do this by activating positive, but realistic, expectations of what can be changed and how. Mental contrasting seems to energize the individual, and then helps them begin to consider strategies for overcoming the obstacles they may face.

Implementation intentions

Further on in the goal-directed process, research has focused on the nature and value of *implementation intentions* (Gollwitzer, 1999; Park-Stamms & Gollwitzer, 2009). This refers to an if-then plan that the individual holds for responding to a particular concrete situation in a particular way. For example, a client who wants to develop her self-confidence might say, 'If my colleague at work puts me down, I will ask him not to do that again'. Research indicates that implementation intentions are a highly effective means of supporting goal attainment, with research across 94 independent studies showing a medium to large effect size of $d = 0.65$ (Gollwitzer & Sheeran, 2006). By establishing implementation intentions, it is hypothesized that people become more sensitized to when the critical situation is emerging (e.g. recognizing that they are being put down by their colleague), and then automating the initiation of the planned behaviour (e.g. naturally responding in a more assertive way). Interestingly, a consequence of this automization is that implementation intentions seem to be particularly effective when the individual is 'ego depleted' (i.e. mentally tired, Gollwitzer & Sheeran, 2006).

Feedback

'For goals to be effective', write Locke and Latham (Locke & Latham, 2002), 'people need summary feedback that reveals progress in relation to their goals' (p. 708). Consistent with this assertion, meta-analysis has shown that behaviour change interventions which include some element of self-monitoring (e.g. by asking participants to keep an activity diary) have significantly greater impact (Michie, Abraham, Whittington, McAteer, & Gupta, 2009). A study by Polivy *et al.* (1986), for instance, found that people were more able to moderate the amount of chocolate that they ate when they could see the wrappers of the chocolates that they had already eaten, compared with when they threw the wrappers away in a wastebasket. Feedback, argue Locke and Latham, allows the person to adjust the level and direction of their efforts to match what the goal requires. This will allow them to intensify efforts if they feel that they are not progressing, and conserve resources (as well as acknowledge their successes) if they are achieving this goal.

Disengagement

Although goal process models tend to focus on goal engagement, an issue that is also of central importance, particularly to the therapeutic field, is that of goal disengagement (e.g. Heckhausen, Wrosch, & Schulz, 2010). As Joostman and Koole (2009) write, 'disengagement can often be an adaptive response to situations in which further investment of time and resources is in undue proportion to the expected outcomes' (p. 337). In other words, an inability to disengage from goals—for instance, when they have become completed, unattainable, or too resource-intensive—may be associated with psychological difficulties. This may be because the person then has fewer resources to invest in actualizing other important goals. It may also be that they experience persistent and chronic feelings of frustration, loss, and hopelessness. Given that goal disengagement is particularly important when goals are unattainable, there may be an interesting interaction here between goal disengagement processes and the degree to which goals are realistically attainable. More specifically, individuals who set highly unrealistic goals, and are then unable to disengage with them, may be predicted to experience greater psychological distress than individuals who set highly unrealistic goals but can easily disengage. For individuals with realistic goals, however, it might be predicted that those who quickly (and prematurely) disengage from them might experience more difficulties than those with a greater degree of perseverance.

Goals as hierarchically organized

A basic assumption among many theorists and researchers in the goals-related fields is that goals can be conceptualized as existing in a hierarchical structure. This ranges from the highest order life meanings to the most concrete, immediate goals (e.g. Austin & Vancouver, 1996; Carver & Scheier, 1990; Little & Gee, 2007). Much of this is derived from Powers' (1973) *control theory* and its *hierarchy of purposes*. Here, higher order goals can be conceptualized as forming the *reference value* for lower order goals; with lower order goals forming the means by which higher order goals may be obtained. As indicated in Figure 3.1, for instance, an individual may have a highest order goal to experience relatedness (Flannagan, 2010; Ryan & Deci, 2000), and one thing they

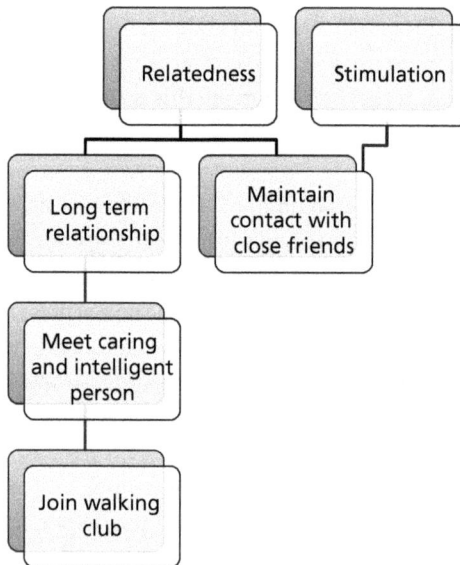

Fig. 3.1 Example hierarchy of goals.

may strive to do to experience this is to establish a long-term relationship. To achieve that, they may try and meet intelligent and caring people and, with that aim in mind, they might plan to join a walking club. These associations between higher order, and lower order, goals are termed vertical relationships, while associations between goals at the same level are termed horizontal relationships (Cooper, 2012).

Although this hierarchical framework posits the existence of highest order goals—or what have been termed 'terminal values' (Austin & Vancouver, 1996; Little & Gee, 2007), 'core projects' (Little, 2007), or 'original projects' (Sartre, 1958)—it leaves open the question of what they might be. Indeed, the framework allows for the possibility that there may be multiple highest order goals (as with, for instance, self-determination theory, Ryan & Deci, 2000), or that no universal set of highest order goals exist—rather, people differ in what they most fundamentally strive for (Cooper & McLeod, 2011). This hierarchical framework also allows for the existential possibility that, ultimately, there are no highest order goals (Camus, 1955; Heidegger, 1962; Sartre, 1958). That is, that while we may strive towards particular goals, ultimately they have no essential foundation: they are self-chosen, meaningless and 'absurd'.

Two principles that are fundamental to these goal hierarchies are those of *equifinality* and *multifinality* (Austin & Vancouver, 1996; Kruglanski & Kopetz, 2009). Equifinality is the principle that the same goal can be achieved through a multiplicity of different lower order goals (Austin & Vancouver, 1996). Hence, for instance, a person may strive to attain relatedness through a long-term relationship, but they may also try and achieve it through maintaining contact with their close friends (see Figure 3.1). A system in which there are high levels of equifinality can be described as flexible, in that an individual can achieve the same goal in multiple different ways (Caspar, 2005). By contrast, a unifinal system will have the quality of rigidity and inflexibility. Multifinality (or 'heterarchy', Austin & Vancouver, 1996) refers to the principle that the same lower order goal may achieve multiple higher order goals. For instance, the desire to spend time with friends may also be a means of achieving stimulation and excitement (see Figure 3.1). Research suggests that people may have an inherent tendency—unconsciously as well as consciously—towards adopting multifinal means (Chun *et al.*, 2011), and this is consistent with a wider belief in an underlying universal tendency towards synergies (Corning, 2003, see below). That is, when all other things are equal, we will choose towards acting in ways that can satisfy multiple goals at one point in time. Such a system, in which there are high levels of multifinality, can be described as *synergistic*, while a system in which there are low levels of multifinality can be described as *dysergetic* (see below) (Cooper, 2012).

From a clinical perspective, one of the key strengths of this goal hierarch-ical framework is that it provides a means of understanding how psychological difficulties may evolve and be maintained. Two intrapersonal mechanisms, in particular, can be highlighted: horizontal incoherence and vertical incoherence (Cooper, 2012; Sheldon & Kasser, 1995) (social and environmental mecha-nisms will be discussed later in the chapter).

Horizontal relationships: synergy and dysergy between goals

As we have seen, across similar levels in a goal hierarchy, multiple goals may exist. Riediger (2007) suggests that three types of relationships that may exist between these goals—*interference, facilitation,* and *independence*—and this is largely consistent with other theorizing in this field (e.g. Little, 1983; Riediger, 2007). Note, research here indicates that goal interference and goal facilitation are independent dimensions, rather than opposite ends of a single dimension (e.g. Boudreaux & Ozer, 2013). That is, two goals can both facilitate each other and interfere with each other. For instance, 'eating nice food' may help someone towards their goal of 'happiness', but it might also work against the latter goal by being an expensive pursuit.

A facilitative relationship between goals means that 'the pursuit of one goal simultaneously increases the likelihood of reaching another goal' (Wiese & Salmela-Aro, 2008, p. 490). This has also been termed *positive spillover* (Wiese & Salmela-Aro, 2008); and, in the language of the wider social sciences field, is synonymous with *synergetic* (Corning, 2003), *non-zero-sum* (Wright, 2000), *win-win*, or *cooperative* (Axelrod, 1984) relationships. For instance, if the close friends of the individual in Figure 3.1 are in a walking club, then by joining such a club, she can facilitate the attainment of contact with them, as well as striving towards her goal of meeting a caring and intelligent man or woman.

Alternatively, the relationship between goals may be *interfering, competing, win-lose,* or what is widely termed *goal conflict* (Austin & Vancouver, 1996; Michalak & Grosse Holtfort, 2006; Wiese & Salmela-Aro, 2008). Here, 'a goal that a person wishes to accomplish interferes with the attainment of at least one other goal that the individual simultaneously wishes to accomplish' (Michalak, Heidenreich, & Hoyer, 2004, p. 84). These goals can also be described as dys-ergetic (Cooper, 2012): the antonym of a synergetic relationship, in which the whole is *less* than the sum of the parts. For instance, it may be that, in trying to establish a long-term relationship, the woman actually ends up spending less time with her close friends.

The concepts of synergy and dysergy form an essential component of a model of wellbeing which understands people as purposeful and agentic. For if human beings are understood as goal-oriented organism, the question is raised as to why they can fail to actualize their goals, and experience the kind of distress described above? Here, the concept of dysergy suggests that human beings can experience feelings of failure, not because they are not goal-oriented beings, but because they are striving to actualize goals that are incompatible with other important things that they want to achieve. A client, for example, may fail in her goal of achieving close relationships with other people, and this may be because she avoids any form of social contact. But this avoidance, itself, can be seen as a goal-oriented form of behaviour: for instance, an attempt to feel safe because she has experienced so much hurt in relationships in the past.

This hypothesis, that goal conflict is a source of psychological distress, is prevalent within the psychological literature (e.g. Kelly, Mansell, & Wood, 2015; Riediger, 2007). Indeed, Powers (1973) writes that 'Since the time of Freud and no doubt for much longer than that, inner conflicts have been recognized as a major cause of psychological difficulties' (p. 265). The hypothesis is supported by empirical research which shows that goal conflict is associated with higher levels of psychological symptoms, and lower levels of psychological function- ing, affect, mobilization, and life satisfaction (Austin & Vancouver, 1996; Cox & Klinger, 2002; Emmons, 1986; Emmons & King, 1988; Karoly, 1999; Kelly *et al.*, 2015; Riediger, 2007; Riediger & Freund, 2004). Summarizing the research, Michalak and colleagues (2004) write: 'most studies reveal a relation between intrapsychic conflicts and people's psychopathological status' (p. 90). As sug- gested, this may be because, where goal conflict exists, people are failing to achieve important goals. Mansell (2005) likens goal conflict to 'two different air conditioning systems operating in the same room, one set at 20°C and the other at 30°C' (p. 147). Here, neither system will ever achieve their goal. However, like two people in the same room trying to regulate according to different tempera- ture goals, the very existence of an internal conflict may also evoke feelings of turmoil, confusion, and disintegration in a person; and may leave them feeling exhausted and drained of resources (Karoly, 1999). This latter explanation, as opposed to the former, is supported by research by Boudreaux and Ozer (2013), which showed that individuals with greater levels of goal conflict were less suc- cessful in achieving their goals, but the ones that they failed to achieve were not necessarily the ones in conflict.

One particular form of dysergetic inter-goal relationship that has been asso- ciated with psychological problems is *arbitrary control* (Mansell, 2005; Powers, 1973). Here, the person acts towards one particular goal or set of goals (the 'active goal', Bargh & Huang, 2009) without regard to the wider goals network. This can be likened to *tunnel vision* or *selective attention*, and is consistent with Bargh and Huang's (2009) theory that goals are essentially 'selfish' and 'will single-mindedly pursue their agenda independently of whether doing so is in the overall good of the individual person' (p. 131). Such autonomous, single-minded forces might be termed *rogue goals*, and could be hypothesized to exist at the core of many maladaptive psychological processes. For instance, a young person gets 'taken over' by the aim of being thin, and neglects the many other goals that are of importance to her, such as being healthy and having friends. In fact, research suggests that people, in general, tend to be quite good at switching to more important, higher order goals when they are tempted by incompatible lower order goals (Heckhausen *et al.*, 2010). However, some people may be more vulnerable to arbitrary control, and this may relate to the existence of meta-goals, such as 'I always want to complete my goals'. Goals that are unconscious may also have more power to exert arbitrary control because the person is less able to stand back from them and consider their wider goals network.

Conversely, it is widely hypothesized in the goals' literature that 'harmony and integrated functioning among one's goals are essential for subjective wellbeing' (Emmons, 1986, p. 1065). Interestingly, however, the evidence here is less compelling, with a number of studies finding no directed relationship between inter-goal facilitation and wellbeing (Riediger, 2007; Wiese & Salmela-Aro, 2008), although other studies have (Sheldon & Kasser, 1995). What does seem clear, however, is that the more synergetic a person's goals, the more the person tends 'to engage in goal directed actions' (Riediger & Freund, 2004, p. 1522). It may also be that it is the ratio of facilitative to interfering inter-goal relationships that is the 'crucial characteristic' of a goal system that facilitates wellbeing (Wiese & Salmela-Aro, 2008).

Vertical relationships: effective and ineffective means

Although the psychological literature has tended to focus on horizontal coherence, Sheldon and Kasser (1995) also highlight the importance of *vertical coherence*: whether or not the subgoals actually help someone progress towards the goals that they are aiming for. Here, 'an action system is optimally configured when purposes at higher levels of the system are readily served by behavioral competencies at lower levels of the system' (Sheldon & Kasser, 1998, p. 1319). For instance, if someone's goal is to meet a partner who is caring, serious, and environmentally aware, joining a walking club may be a very good idea. But the same strategy may be highly ineffective if, for instance, they want to meet a partner who likes staying up all night clubbing. Note, the hypothesis that people are sometimes ineffective in their goal-attainment strategies does not contradict the earlier proposition that people are, inherently, agentic beings who act towards their world in meaningful and intelligible ways. Human beings may strive to 'do their best', but this does not always mean that the thing they think will be best is actually the most effective means of actualizing their goals.

Why might people strive towards their goals in ineffective ways? One reason may be simply learning: for instance, a person may not have learnt yet that members of walking clubs do not tend to like all night clubbing. We may also choose to adopt strategies that were effective in past times, but are no longer so. For instance, a person might have learnt, as a child, that the best way to get their need for love and attention met was by being very compliant and submissive and, as an adult, they continue with this strategy, even though this now elicits a more rejecting response. A third possibility is that the person's higher order goals are unconscious (see above), and therefore they cannot work towards them effectively. For instance, if what I deeply want from a relationship is to feel unconditionally loved, but do not recognize this (or think that I want something else, such as sex or status), then I am unlikely to develop strategies (e.g. expressing my vulnerabilities) that may best help me achieve my goals.

Hierarchy of goals as a unifying theoretical framework

This hierarchical model of goals provides a useful means of drawing together many of the goal-related concepts and processes discussed earlier. Goals that are long-term, abstract, and more important can be understood as higher order goals; whereas short-term, concrete, and less important goals can be understood as lower down in the hierarchy of goals. In addition, with the concepts of arbitrary control and rogue goals, we can see how lower level goals may, at times, take over, and why this may not serve the person as a whole. Goals may be approach or avoidant at any level in the hierarchy; but we can understand intrinsic goals as those closely related to the highest order goals, while extrinsic goals can be understood as lower down the hierarchy, and particularly a sub-branch of the desire for approval (Cooper, 2013). This would explain why progress towards extrinsic goals is less likely to bring about positive affect than intrinsic goals: it has less of a direct impact on our highest order desires, and it is also more contingent on factors that are outside of an individual's own control. Within this framework, there is the possibility that goals at any level can be conscious or unconscious. However, as discussed above, the more conscious goals are, the more empowered individuals are to develop synergetic and effective methods to achieve these goals, and to draw on such strategies as mental contrasting and implementation intentions.

This hierarchical framework is also consistent with, and capable of encompassing, a wide range of psychotherapeutic models of human functioning (see, Cooper, 2012). The humanistic notion of an actualizing tendency (Rogers, 1959), for instance, can be conceptualized as the tendency of the organismic system towards synergetic configurations, while incongruence (the primary source of pathology in the humanistic model) can be understood as a conflict between intrinsically and extrinsically oriented goals (Cooper, 2013). Existential models are compatible with a concept of the organism as goal-oriented and striving for meaning (e.g. Frankl, 1986). The concept of conflict across motivational system encompasses psychodynamic understandings of the aetiology of psychological distress (Curtis & Hirsch, 2003; Wolitzky, 2003). In the classical Freudian model, for instance, the *id*'s unconscious desire for hedonistic gratification comes up against the *superego*'s desire for moral and socially sanctioned behaviour, with the *ego* that part of the person attempting to achieve mediation and balance (Magnavita, 2008). In cognitive therapy, the many biases and heurisms that people enact can be seen as a manifestation of short-term, rogue goals and temptations (for instance, to avoid 'ego depletion', Moskowitz & Grant, 2009b), which then have the consequence of undermining the organism as a whole. Cognitive and behavioural approaches are also based on the assumption that people often adopt ineffective strategies to achieve their goals, hence the need for such interventions as psychoeducation and assertiveness training (Sanchez, Lewinsohn, & Larson, 1980).

The hierarchical approach presented here also provides a common framework for bringing together a wide range of therapeutic practices. Essentially, what all therapies can be seen as doing is to help people find better ways of actualizing their highest order goals. This may be through supporting people to become more aware, and accepting, of what those highest order goals are; helping people to recognize, reflect on, and resolve conflicts across goals; or teaching people skills that can help them attain the most common higher order goals more effectively. Here, the barriers between different therapeutic orientations can be seen as dissolving: all therapists can be seen as working towards the same goal, albeit with different foci.

The social context

Within the psychological literature, as reviewed above, there is a tendency to focus on goals, goal processes, and inter-goal relationships *within* the person (although see Cavallo & Fitzsimons, 2012; Deci & Ryan, 2012; Heckhausen *et al.*, 2010). Therapeutic models, too, have tended to understand the relationship between goal actualization and psychological distress at the individual level alone (see above) (Cooper, 2015). However, if goals are understood as having an intrinsically in-the-world component, as well as a psychological one (see Chapter 1, this volume), then the extent to which people actualize their goals will also be fundamentally determined by their social environment.

Social factors can determine goals, and goal-related processes, in many ways. First, the kinds of goals that people adopt—right up to their highest order goals (Heidegger, 1962)—are likely to be learnt from their social and cultural environments. Indeed, 'there is research to suggest that goal pursuit is automatically triggered when goals are inferred from the behavior of others' (Aarts & Custers, 2012, p. 235), a process known as 'goal contagion'. In addition, the social context is likely to determine how attainable goals may seem, as well as the extent to which people can actually progress towards, and achieve, them. For instance, an affluent individual, compared with a less affluent one, may feel more able to attain their goal of travelling around the world, and may also be more likely to actually do it. The social context may also play a key role in determining the extent to which goals come into conflict with each other (Cooper, 2012, 2016). As I have argued (Cooper, 2006):

> [O]ur wants are often in tension with each other ... because we inhabit an environment in which the achievement of one want frequently necessitates the subjugation of another. A person in a context of limited financial resources, for example, might only be able to achieve their desire for financial security by suppressing their desire for excitement and stimulation: for instance, by taking a job in a fast food restaurant. Alternatively, in that environment, the person may be able to actualise their desire for stimulation by forming a musical group with their friends, but then they might have to compromise their desire for financial security. (p. 88)

From this standpoint, then, conflict arises between a person's goal because of *limited resources* in their context (Boudreaux & Ozer, 2013; Michalak *et al.*, 2004; Riediger & Freund, 2004). This is an individual-level equivalent to social psychology's *realistic conflict theory*, which holds that 'limited resources lead to conflict among groups' (Aronson, Wilson, & Akert, 1999, p. 486).

Given, as discussed above, the relationship between goal actualization and positive affect, this framework shows how social factors, as well as psychological ones, may influence our levels of wellbeing and distress. An individual who is rich enough, for instance, to go travelling around the world, and who is able to actually finance such a trip, is likely to experience more goal actualization—and therefore more positive affect—than an individual without such resources. This is consistent with research which shows that social factors, such as poverty and political oppression, can reduce levels of positive affect (Wilkinson & Pickett, 2010).

Implications for setting goals in therapy

This review of the psychological literature on goals and goal processes suggests that there is a wealth of theory and evidence on which therapists can draw for their practice. This final section aims to draw out some of these implications, with specific reference to setting goals in therapy.

Goal-setting may be undertaken with clients in a relatively informal and 'low-key' way. For instance, it may simply involve asking clients about the things that they want in therapy, and keeping a mental note of this as the therapeutic work progresses. On the other hand, it may take a more formal and prominent form: particularly through the use of written goal-based measures and instruments (see Chapter 6, this volume) (Hurn, Kneebone, & Cropley, 2006). Through completing forms such as the goal-based outcome measure (Law & Jacob, 2015), or through processes such as personal projects analysis (Little & Gee, 2007), clients can be explicitly encouraged to reflect on, and reconsider, their personal goals. And, indeed, there are not only tools to help clients identify their goals, but also to consider the levels of conflict and synergy between them (e.g. the Striving Instrumentality Matrix, Emmons & King, 1988). Asking clients to formally record their goals may support the goal actualization process by helping them to develop clearer and more specific formulations of their goals, it can remind clients of what their important goals are, and it can provide feedback on goal progress. However, the downside of formal goal-setting is that it may inhibit the client from revising or reconceptualizing their goals as the therapeutic work progresses.

So is it useful to set goals for therapy, either formally or informally? Generally, research from the psychological field would suggest it is: that encouraging both adults and children to set goals has the capacity to facilitate their attainment (Locke & Latham, 2002; Schunk, 1990), and is generally linked to higher levels of wellbeing (Aked, 2008). Locke and Latham (2002), in their analysis of the evidence, suggest that there are a range of reasons for this. First, focusing on goals helps to direct people's attention and effort on goal-related activities, and away from activities that are unrelated to that goal. Second, setting goals can help energize people towards goal-directed action. Third, by having goals, people may be more likely to be persistent. Fourth, having goals can lead to the arousal and discovery of task-relevant knowledge and strategies.

Within a therapeutic context, the process of setting goals also may be important because it can help clients to become more aware of unconscious goals. This may be helpful for a number of reasons. First, it may help clients feel more in control, and more understanding and accepting of themselves. Moreover, by becoming more conscious of their goals, the individual can explore alternative, and potentially more effective, means of actualizing them. They can also reflect on, and reconsider, whether these are the goals and subgoals that they want to strive towards; and look at ways of overcoming goal conflict and arbitrary control (Mansell, 2005). Hence, conscious elicitation and exploration allows clients to direct their attention to their overall goals hierarchy, and to reconfigure their ways of doing things to optimize their actualization of highest order goals.

However, there may also be limits to the value of goal-setting in therapy and, in some instances, it may have the potential to be counter-therapeutic. This could be for a number of reasons. First, the setting of goals is only likely to be salutogenic to the extent that the goals are helpful ones to pursue. A client, for instance, who sets for themselves avoidant, extrinsic goals (for instance, 'I don't want people to think I'm a fool'), may be helped in their achievement, but this may do little for the client's overall wellbeing. Second, given the levels of incongruence between people's self-identified motives and their intrinsic goals, there is a danger that clients' explicitly set therapeutic goals will bear little relation to their actual, highest order desires. This might make elements of the therapeutic work redundant and mean that the time and resources of the therapist and client are being diverted down 'blind alleys' that will satisfy only the most superficial of goals. Goal-setting in therapy, then, is only likely to be helpful to the extent that the client's self-identified goals match their intrinsic ones. This means that goal-setting may be most helpful to clients who have such qualities as self-determination and sensitivity to bodily states (see Thrash *et al.*, 2012, discussed above). It also means that, in any goal-setting process, there should be time for clients to reflect on their higher order goals and desires, and to be able to revise them as 'emergent goals' appear in the client's consciousness (John McLeod, personal communication, 24 August 2016). It also means that therapists should explore with their clients what their goals mean and 'unpack' them, rather than simply taking them at face-value. Third, research suggests that, while a majority of clients do want to set goals in therapy, there are a significant minority who do not (Cooper & Norcross, 2015). This may be related to clients' meta-goals: for instance, a client may be striving to get away from fixed and demanding goals in her life. Although, of course, this is a goal in itself, given the evidence that clients do better in therapies that match their preferences (Swift, Callahan, & Vollmer, 2011), it is likely to be counter-therapeutic (as well as unethical) to impose a goal-setting process on such clients.

Nevertheless, given that some clients are likely to find explicit goal-setting helpful at some points in therapy, what are the characteristics of a 'well-formed therapeutic goal' (see also Grosse Holtforth & Michalak, 2012, and Chapter 7, this volume). Based on this review of the evidence, we can suggest it is likely to have the following qualities:

- *Intrinsic*: Clearly and directly related to higher order needs—such as connectedness, autonomy, or a sense of community—rather than contingent on the attitudes or actions of others. In working with children and young people, it may also be important to set goals that are intrinsic and meaningful to *them*, as opposed to the adults that may have brought the children to therapy.

- *Effective*: A credible means of attaining higher order goals, rather than an inefficient or indirect strategy. Therapists should also be mindful of meta-goals (including affect- and competence-related goals), that may trigger vicious downward spirals.

- *Synergetic*: Supportive of other therapeutic goals or, at least, not in conflict with them (an example of the latter might be 'I want more time on my own', when the client has already stated 'I want to be closer to my partner'). Therapists should be particularly mindful of rogue goals, which are focused on actualizing just one part of the person to the detriment of the greater whole.

- *Approach*: About achieving something positive, rather than avoiding something negative.

- *Challenging*: 'Stretching' for the person …

- *Realistic*: … but realistically achievable within the therapeutic time frame. Goals that come from clients' unrealistically high expectations of themselves (for instance, 'I want to feel calm all the time') should be challenged. Therapists should also be mindful of the number of goals that clients are setting: are there too many to be realistically achieved (or too few to be sufficiently challenging)? If, as the work proceeds, it becomes apparent that clients' goals are unattainable, it may be important to support them in the process of disengaging.

- *Important*: Clients are likely to experience a greater sense of accomplishment if they can work towards important goals. However, if clients are struggling to attain any goals (as might be the case with children), it may be better for them to begin by setting, and attaining, relatively unimportant goals (hence boosting their self-efficacy), rather than striving for, and failing to actualize, more important goals.

- *Specific*: Clients may be more able to achieve specific, concrete, and simple goals (e.g. 'Talk back to my bully at work') over vague, abstract, and complex ones (e.g. 'Be assertive'). However, this needs to be weighed against the relative importance of these goals and their proximity to higher order goals. An optimal goal is probably both specific and also relatively high order (e.g. 'Share more about myself with my closest friends').

- *Supported with mental contrasting and implementation intentions*: There is evidence that both these processes can facilitate the attainment of goals. Clients should be encouraged to think about what they are aiming for, how this contrasts with their current situation, and to develop concrete plans for progressing from 'A' to 'B'.

- *Supported with feedback*: Regular monitoring of goal attainment, whether informally or through more structured goal attainment measures, seems to be of benefit.

◆ *Mindful of the social context:* Clients' goals, and their capacity to actualize them, are likely to be dependent on their social, cultural, interpersonal, and political context. These factors must be borne in mind in terms of what might make attainable goals, and also where the points of leverage may be in achieving them.

Implications for therapeutic formulations

Although less developed, the evidence and framework reviewed in this chapter can also serve as the basis for developing an understanding of clients and their psychological difficulties. Caspar (2005), for instance, has developed a model of formulation, 'plan analysis', which maps out clients' goals and subgoals in hierarchical format, to develop an understanding of the problems that have brought them into therapy, and the kind of therapeutic relationship that may be of greatest value to them. Such a hierarchical analysis may be helpful to therapists of any orientation. In addition, in understanding the source of clients' difficulties, therapists may find it useful to ask themselves the following questions at the formulation stage:

◆ Does my client have a sense of what they are striving for in life?

◆ Does my client see their goals as attainable?

◆ Does my client feel that they are moving towards their goals, and is this at a fast enough pace?

◆ Has my client achieved important goals in their life?

◆ Are the things that my client is striving towards actually important to them?

◆ Are my clients' goals sufficiently challenging?

◆ Is my client oriented towards approach goals, or avoidance goals?

◆ Are my clients' predominant goals intrinsically satisfying to them, or are they linked to earning praise from others?

◆ Are my client's goals specific?

◆ Does my client have goals that are in the near future, or are they all in the distant future?

◆ Is my client aware of the things that they are most deeply striving for in life?

◆ What are my client's meta-goals: their goals about their goal striving?

◆ Does my client compare past with future, to get a sense of how to move from one to the other, or do they unproductively fantasize about the future or dwell in the past?

◆ Does my client have specific if-then strategies for overcoming obstacles in their goal pursuits?

- Does my client have ways of monitoring how well they are progressing towards their goals?
- Is my client able to disengage from unattainable goals?
- Are my client's predominant goals in conflict, or are they facilitative of each other?
- Does my client have any rogue goals?
- Does my client have effective means of achieving their goals?
- Are my client's goals achievable within their social and interpersonal circumstances? Do they need to change these circumstances to achieve their goals?

Implications for therapeutic practice

The analysis developed in this chapter does not propose a new way of doing therapy. Rather, as suggested earlier, it provides a framework for drawing together a wide variety of therapeutic practices, and underscoring some key principles of practice. These can be briefly summarized as follows:

- help clients become more aware of what it is that they really want in life: what their highest order, most intrinsic goals are;
- help clients reflect on what stops getting them to these goals, and how they might go about doing things more effectively;
- help clients look at goals that might be in conflict with each other, and how they could go about creating more synergetic inter-goal relationships.

In addition, as part of the ongoing therapeutic dialogue, clients can be encouraged to explore all of the questions articulated above in the 'Implications for therapeutic formulations' section of this chapter, as and where relevant. This may help them develop their own understanding of how their problems may have evolved, as well as potential solutions. For instance, at relevant places in the therapeutic dialogue, clients might be encouraged to consider whether they are sufficiently able to disengage from unattainable goals, whether their goals are approach- or avoidance-oriented, or whether they have if-then plans for achieving particular goals. This can then support clients to find more effective ways towards goal actualization.

Conclusion

Given the evidence presented in this chapter, there is no doubt that the process of applying psychological evidence on goals to therapeutic practice must be done in a sensitive and thoughtful way. As we have seen, for instance, principles of helpful goal-setting can come into conflict with each other: challenging but realistic goals, specific but important, balancing levels of engagement and disengagement. Moreover, given that many of the clients' highest order goals are at an unconscious, latent level, the therapeutic process becomes a complex, evolving dance among setting, acting on, working with, and re-evaluating goals. Nevertheless, psychological theory and research on goals and goal processes is a vast, untapped reservoir of knowledge on which clinicians can draw to enhance their therapeutic work. In the psychological field, there is clear evidence that goal-oriented activities, of particular types, can be salutogenic. Applied to the clinical context—with appropriate testing, evaluation, and development—these have the potential to make a major contribution to the enhancement of therapeutic practice.

Points for reflection

◆ Identify three goals that are of particular importance to you at the present moment. Now consider the extent to which your current wellbeing is related to your actualization of these goals (for instance, experiencing them as attainable, progressing towards them).

◆ For each of the three goals identified above, also consider where they lie on each of the dimensions outlined in the second part of this chapter (e.g. importance, challenge, approach vs. avoidance). You may also find it useful to consider how a client might respond to these questions.

◆ What do you think are the most important principles that can be derived from the literature reviewed here on how to work with goals and goal processes in clinical practice?

Acknowledgements

Thanks to Sarah Cantwell, Duncan Law, John McLeod, and Joel Vos for invaluable feedback on an earlier draft of this chapter.

Further reading

Austin, J. T., & Vancouver, J. B. (1996). Goal constructs in psychology: Structure, process, and content. *Psychological Bulletin, 120*(3), 338–75.
Still, probably, the most comprehensive review paper of the goals literature in psychology.
Little, B. R., Salmela-Aro, K., & Phillips, S. D. (Eds.). (2007). *Personal project pursuit: Goals, action, and human flourishing.* Mahwah, NJ: Lawrence Erlbaum Associates Publishers.
Valuable collection of chapters on all aspects of goals-related practice.
Moskowitz, G. B., & Grant, H. (Eds.). (2009). *The psychology of goals.* New York: Guilford Press.
Rich and in-depth collection of chapters on the psychology of goals, with a particular focus on the motivation-cognition relationship. See also Aarts and Elliot (2012) which has a similar range of chapters.

Grosse Holtfort, M., & Michalak, J. (2012). Motivation in psychotherapy. In R. M. Ryan (Ed.), *The Oxford handbook of human motivation* (pp. 441–462). New York: Oxford University Press.

Valuable review of the evidence on goals and goal-setting in relation to therapeutic practice.

References

Aarts, H., & Custers, R. (2012). Unconscious goal pursuit: Nonconscious goal regulation and motivation. In R. M. Ryan (Ed.), *The Oxford handbook of human motivation* (pp. 232–47). New York: Oxford University Press.

Ajzen, I. (1991). The theory of planned behavior. *Organizational behavior and human decision processes, 50*(2), 179–211.

Aked, J., Marks, N., Cordon, C., & Thompson, S. (2008). *Five ways to wellbeing: The evidence*. London: nef.

Aronson, E., Wilson, T. D., & Akert, R. M. (1999). *Social Psychology*. New York: Longman.

Austin, J. T., & Vancouver, J. B. (1996). Goal constructs in psychology: Structure, process, and content. *Psychological Bulletin, 120*(3), 338–75. doi: 10.1037/0033-2909.120.3.338

Axelrod, R. (1984). *The evolution of cooperation*. New York: Basic.

Bargh, J. A. (1990). Auto-motives: Preconscious determinants of thought and behavior. Multiple affects from multiple stages. In E. T. Higgins & R. M. Sorrentino (Eds.), *Handbook of motivation and cognition: Foundations of social behavior* (Vol. 2, pp. 93–130). New York: Guilford.

Bargh, J. A., & Ferguson, M. J. (2000). Beyond behaviorism: On the automaticity of higher mental processes. *Psychological Bulletin, 126*(6), 925–45. doi: 10.1037/0033-2909.126.6.925

Bargh, J. A., Gollwitzer, P. M., Lee-Chai, A., Barndollar, K., & Trötschel, R. (2001). The automated will: Nonconscious activation and pursuit of behavioral goals. *Journal of Personality and Social Psychology, 81*(6), 1014–27. doi: 10.1037/0022-3514.81.6.1014

Bargh, J. A., & Huang, J. Y. (2009). The selfish goal. In G. B. Moskowitz & H. Grant (Eds.), *The psychology of goals* (pp. 127–150). New York: Guilford Press.

Berking, M., Grosse Holtforth, M., Jacobi, C., & Kröner-Herwig, B. (2005). Empirically based guidelines for goal-finding procedures in psychotherapy: Are some goals easier to attain than others? *Psychotherapy Research, 15*(3), 316–24. doi: 10.1080/10503300500091801

Boudreaux, M. J., & Ozer, D. J. (2013). Goal conflict, goal striving, and psychological well-being. *Motivation and Emotion, 37*(3), 433–43.

Brunstein, J. C. (1993). Personal goals and subjective well-being: A longitudinal study. *Journal of Personality and Social Psychology, 65*(5), 1061–70. doi: 10.1037/0022-3514.65.5.1061

Camus, A. (1955). *The Myth of Sisyphus* (J. O'Brien, Trans.). London: Penguin.

Carver, C. S., & Scheier, M. F. (1990). Origins and functions of positive and negative affect: A control-process view. *Psychological Review, 97*(1), 19–35. doi: 10.1037/0033-295x.97.1.19

Carver, C. S., & Scheier, M. F. (2012). Cybernetic control processes and the self-regulation of behavior. In R. M. Ryan (Ed.), *The Oxford handbook of human motivation* (pp. 28–42). New York: Oxford University Press.

Caspar, F. (2005). *Plan analysis: Towards optimizing psychotherapy.* Bern: Hogrefe & Huber.

Cavallo, J. V., & Fitzsimons, G. M. (2012). Goal competition, conflict, coordination, and completion: How intergoal dynamics affect self-regulation. In H. Aarts & A. J. Elliot (Eds.), *Goal-directed behavior* (pp. 267–300). New York: Psychology Press.

Chun, W. Y., Kruglanski, A. W., Sleeth-Keppler, D., & Friedman, R. S. (2011). Multifinality in implicit choice. *Journal of Personality and Social Psychology, 101*(5), 1124–37.

Cooper, M. (2006). Socialist humanism: A progressive politics for the twenty-first century. In G. Proctor, M. Cooper, P. Sanders & B. Malcolm (Eds.), *Politicising the Person-Centred Approach: An Agenda for Social Change* (pp. 80–94). Ross-on-Wye: PCCS Books.

Cooper, M. (2012). *A hierarchy of wants: Towards an integrative framework for counselling, psychotherapy and social change.* University of Strathclyde. Glasgow. Retrieved from download from pure.strath.ac.uk/portal

Cooper, M. (2013). The intrinsic foundations of extrinsic motivations and goals: Towards a unified humanistic theory of wellbeing. *Journal of Humanistic Psychology, 53*(2), 153–71. doi: 10.1177/0022167812453768

Cooper, M. (2015). Social change from the counselling room. *Therapy Today, 26*(2), 10–13.

Cooper, M. (2016). The fully functioning society: A humanistic-existential vision of an actualizing, socially-just future. *Journal of Humanistic Psychology.* doi: 10.1177/0022167816659755

Cooper, M., & Joseph, S. (2016). Psychological foundations for humanistic psychotherapeutic practice. In D. Cain, K. Keenan & S. Rubin (Eds.), *Humanistic psychotherapies* (2nd ed., pp. 11–46). Washington: APA.

Cooper, M., & McLeod, J. (2011). *Pluralistic Counselling and Psychotherapy.* London: Sage.

Cooper, M., & Norcross, J. C. (2015). A Brief, Multidimensional Measure of Clients' Therapy Preferences: The Cooper-Norcross Inventory of Preferences (C-NIP). *International Journal of Clinical and Health Psychology, 16*(1). doi: 10.1016/j.ijchp.2015.08.003

Corning, P. (2003). *Nature's magic: Synergy in evolution and the fate of humankind.* Cambridge: Cambridge University.

Cox, W. M., & Klinger, E. (2002). Motivational structure: Relationships with substance use and processes of change. *Addictive Behaviors, 27*(6), 925–40. doi: 10.1016/S0306-4603(02)00290-3

Curtis, R. C., & Hirsch, I. (2003). Relational approaches to psychoanalytic psychotherapy. In A. S. Gurman & S. B. Messer (Eds.), *Essential Psychotherapies: Theory and Practice* (2nd ed., pp. 69–106). New York: Guilford Press.

Deci, E. L., & Ryan, R. M. (2012). Motivation, personality, and development within embedded social contexts: An overview of self-determination theory. In R. M. Ryan (Ed.), *The Oxford handbook of human motivation* (pp. 85–107). New York: Oxford University Press.

Dweck, C. S., & Leggett, E. L. (1988). A social-cognitive approach to motivation and personality. *Psychological review, 95*(2), 256.

Elliot, A. J., & Church, M. A. (2002). Client articulated avoidance goals in the therapy context. *Journal of Counseling Psychology, 49*(2), 243–54. doi: 10.1037/0022-0167.49.2.243

Elliot, A. J., & Friedman, R. (2007). Approach-avoidance: A central characteristic of personal goals. In B. R. Little, K. Salmela-Aro & S. D. Phillips (Eds.), *Personal project pursuit: Goals, action, and human flourishing.* (pp. 97–118). Mahwah, NJ: Lawrence Erlbaum Associates Publishers.

Elliot, A. J., & Sheldon, K. M. (1997). Avoidance achievement motivation: a personal goals analysis. *Journal of Personality and Social Psychology, 73*(1), 171.

Elliott, E. S., & Dweck, C. S. (1988). Goals: an approach to motivation and achievement. *Journal of Personality and Social Psychology, 54*(1), 5.

Emmons, R. A. (1986). Personal strivings: An approach to personality and subjective well-being. *Journal of Personality and Social Psychology, 51*(5), 1058–68. doi: 10.1037/0022-3514.51.5.1058

Emmons, R. A., & Diener, E. (1986). A goal-affect analysis of everyday situational choices. *Journal of Research in Personality, 20*(3), 309–26.

Emmons, R. A., & King, L. A. (1988). Conflict among personal strivings: Immediate and long-term implications for psychological and physical well-being. *Journal of Personality and Social Psychology, 54*(6), 1040–8. doi: 10.1037/0022-3514.54.6.1040

Flannagan, C. M. (2010). The case for needs in psychotherapy. *Journal of Psychotherapy Integration, 20*(1), 1–36.

Ford, M. E., & Nichols, C. W. (1987). A taxonomy of human goals and some possible applications. In M. E. Ford & D. H. Ford (Eds.), *Humans as self-constructing living systems: Putting the framework to work* (pp. 289–311). Hillsdale, NJ: Erlbaum.

Frankl, V. E. (1984). *Man's Search for Meaning* (revised and updated ed.). New York: Washington Square Press.

Frankl, V. E. (1986). *The Doctor and the Soul: From Psychotherapy to Logotherapy* (R. Winston & C. Winston, Trans. 3rd ed.). New York: Vintage Books.

Freund, A. M., Hennecke, M., & Mustafic, M. (2012). On gains and losses, means and ends: Goal orientation and goal focus across adulthood. In R. M. Ryan (Ed.), *The Oxford handbook of human motivation* (pp. 280–300). New York: Oxford University Press.

Fujita, K., & MacGregor, K. E. (2012). Basic goal distinctions. In H. Aarts & A. J. Elliot (Eds.), *Goal-directed behavior* (pp. 85–114). New York: Psychology Press.

Gollwitzer, P. M. (1990). Action phases and mind-sets. *Handbook of motivation and cognition: Foundations of social behavior, 2*, 53–92.

Gollwitzer, P. M. (1999). Implementation intentions: strong effects of simple plans. *American Psychologist, 54*(7), 493.

Gollwitzer, P. M., & Oettingen, G. (2012). Goal pursuit. In R. M. Ryan (Ed.), *The Oxford handbook of human motivation* (pp. 208–231). New York: Oxford University Press.

Gollwitzer, P. M., & Sheeran, P. (2006). Implementation intentions and goal achievement: A meta-analysis of effects and processes. *Advances in Experimental Social Psychology, 38*, 69–119.

Grosse Holtforth, M., & Michalak, J. (2012). Motivation in psychotherapy. In R. M. Ryan (Ed.), *The Oxford handbook of human motivation* (pp. 441–462). New York: Oxford University Press.

Grouzet, F. M. E., Kasser, T., Ahuvia, A., Dols, J. M. F., Kim, Y., Lau, S., Ryan, R.M., Saunders, S., Schmuck, P., Sheldon, K. M. (2005). The Structure of Goal Contents Across 15 Cultures. *Journal of Personality and Social Psychology, 89*(5), 800–16. doi: 10.1037/0022-3514.89.5.800

Hanley, T., Sefi, A., & Ersahin, Z. (2015). From goals to tasks and methods. In M. Cooper & W. Dryden (Eds.), *Handbook of pluralistic counselling and psychotherapy* (pp. 28–41). London: Sage.

Heckhausen, H., & Gollwitzer, P. M. (1987). Thought contents and cognitive functioning in motivational versus volitional states of mind. *Motivation and Emotion, 11*(2), 101–20.

Heckhausen, J., Wrosch, C., & Schulz, R. (2010). A motivational theory of life-span development. *Psychological Review, 117*(1), 32–60. doi: 10.1037/a0017668

Heidegger, M. (1962). *Being and Time* (J. Macquarrie & E. Robinson, Trans.). Oxford: Blackwell.

Higgins, E. T. (1997). Beyond pleasure and pain. *American Psychologist, 52*(12), 1280.

Holtforth, M. G., & Grawe, K. (2002). Bern inventory of treatment goals: Part 1. Development and first application of a taxonomy of treatment goal themes. *Psychotherapy Research, 12*(1), 79–99.

Hurn, J., Kneebone, I., & Cropley, M. (2006). Goal setting as an outcome measure: a systematic review. *Clinical Rehabilitation, 20*(9), 756–72. doi: 10.1177/0269215506070793

Jacob, J., Edbrooke-Childs, J., Holley, S., Law, D., & Wolpert, M. (2016). Horses for courses? A qualitative exploration of goals formulated in mental health settings by young people, parents, and clinicians. *Clinical Child Psychology and Psychiatry, 21*(2), 208–223.

Joostman, N. B., & Koole, S. L. (2009). When persistence is futile: A functional analysis of action orientation and goal disengagement. In G. B. Moskowitz & H. Grant (Eds.), *The psychology of goals* (pp. 337–361). New York: Guilford Press.

Kahneman, D. (2011). *Thinking, fast and slow*. London: Penguin.

Karoly, P. (1999). A goal systems–self-regulatory perspective on personality, psychopathology, and change. *Review of General Psychology, 3*(4), 264–91. doi: 10.1037/1089-2680.3.4.264

Kasser, T., & Ryan, R. M. (1993). A dark side of the American dream: Correlates of financial success as a central life aspiration. *Journal of Personality and Social Psychology, 65*(2), 410–22. doi: 10.1037/0022-3514.65.2.410

Kasser, T., & Ryan, R. M. (1996). Further examining the American dream: Differential correlates of intrinsic and extrinsic goals. *Personality and Social Psychology Bulletin, 22*(3), 280–7. doi: 10.1177/0146167296223006

Kasser, T., & Ryan, R. M. (2001). Be careful what you wish for: Optimal functioning and the relative attainment of instrinsic and extrinsic goals. In P. Schmuck & K. M. Sheldon (Eds.), *Life goals and well-being: Towards a positive psychology of human striving* (pp. 116–131). Gottingen: Hogrefe & Huber.

Kelly, R. E., Mansell, W., & Wood, A. M. (2015). Goal conflict and well-being: A review and hierarchical model of goal conflict, ambivalence, self-discrepancy and self-concordance. *Personality and Individual Differences, 85*, 212–29.

King, L. A., & Hicks, J. A. (2013). Positive affect and meaning in life. In P. T. P. Wong (Ed.), *The human quest for meaning: Theories, research, and applications* (2nd ed., pp. 125–141). New York: Routledge.

Koestner, R., Lekes, N., Powers, T. A., & Chicoine, E. (2002). Attaining personal goals: Self-concordance plus implementation intentions equals success. *Journal of Personality and Social Psychology, 83*(1), 231–44. doi: 10.1037/0022-3514.83.1.231

Kruglanski, A. W., & Kopetz, C. (2009). What is so special (and nonspecial) about goals?: A view from the cognitive perspective. In G. B. Moskowitz & H. Grant (Eds.), *The psychology of goals* (pp. 27–55). New York: Guilford Press.

Law, D., & Jacob, J. (2015). *Goals and Goal Based Outcomes (GBOs): Some Useful Information* (3rd ed.). London: CAMHS Press at EBPU.

Little, B. R. (1983). Personal projects: A rationale and method for investigation. *Environment and Behavior, 15*(3), 273–309. doi: 10.1177/0013916583153002

Little, B. R. (2007). Prompt and circumstance: The generative contexts of personal projects analysis. In B. R. Little, K. Salmela-Aro & S. D. Phillips (Eds.), *Personal project pursuit: Goals, action, and human flourishing.* (pp. 3–49). Mahwah, NJ: Lawrence Erlbaum Associates Publishers.

Little, B. R., & Gee, T. L. (2007). The methodology of personal projects analysis: Four modules and a funnel. In B. R. Little, K. Salmela-Aro & S. D. Phillips (Eds.), *Personal project pursuit: Goals, action, and human flourishing.* (pp. 51–94). Mahwah, NJ: Lawrence Erlbaum Associates Publishers.

Little, B. R., Salmela-Aro, K., & Phillips, S. D. (Eds.). (2007). *Personal project pursuit: Goals, action, and human flourishing.* Mahwah, NJ: Lawrence Erlbaum Associates Publishers.

Locke, E. A., & Latham, G. P. (2002). Building a practically useful theory of goal setting and task motivation—A 35-year odyssey. *American Psychologist, 57*(9), 705–717. doi: 10.1037//0003-066x.57.9.705

Mackrill, T. (2011). Differentiating life goals and therapeutic goals. *British Journal of Guidance & Counselling, 39*(1), 25–39.

Magnavita, J. J. (2008). Psychoanalytic psychotherapy. In J. LeBow (Ed.), *Twenty-First Century Psychotherapies: Contemporary Approaches to Theory and Practice* (pp. 206–36). London: Wiley.

Mansell, W. (2005). Control theory and psychopathology: An integrative approach. [doi:10.1348/147608304 X21400]. *Psychology and Psychotherapy: Theory, Research and Practice, 78,* 141–78.

Marien, H., Custers, R., Hassin, R. R., & Aarts, H. (2012). Unconscious goal activation and the hijacking of the executive function. *Journal of Personality and Social Psychology, 103*(3), 399.

McClelland, D. C., Koestner, R., & Weinberger, J. (1989). How do self-attributed and implicit motives differ? *Psychological Review, 96*(4), 690.

Mcleod, J. (2012). What do clients want from therapy? A practice-friendly review of research into client preferences. *European Journal of Psychotherapy and Counselling, 14*(1), 19–32.

Michalak, J., & Grosse Holtfort, M. (2006). Where Do We Go From Here? The Goal Perspective in Psychotherapy. *Clinical Psychology: Science and Practice, 13*(4), 346–65.

Michalak, J., Heidenreich, T., & Hoyer, J. (2004). Goal conflicts: Concepts, findings, and consequences for psychotherapy. In W. M. Cox & E. Klinger (Eds.), *Handbook of Motivational Counseling* (pp. 83–97). New York: John Wiley.

Michie, S., Abraham, C., Whittington, C., McAteer, J., & Gupta, S. (2009). Effective techniques in healthy eating and physical activity interventions: a meta-regression. *Health Psychology, 28*(6), 690.

Moskowitz, G. B., & Grant, H. (2009a). Introduction: Four themes in the study of goals. In G. B. Moskowitz & H. Grant (Eds.), *The psychology of goals* (pp. 1–24). New York: Guilford Press.

Moskowitz, G. B., & Grant, H. (Eds.). (2009b). *The psychology of goals.* New York: Guilford Press.

Murayama, K., Elliot, A. J., & Friedman, R. (2012). Achievement goals. In R. M. Ryan (Ed.), *The Oxford handbook of human motivation* (pp. 191–207). New York: Oxford University Press.

Oettingen, G., & Stephens, E. J. (2009). Fantasies and motivationally intelligent goal setting. In G. B. Moskowitz & H. Grant (Eds.), *The psychology of goals* (pp. 153–78). New York: Guilford Press.

Park-Stamms, E. J., & Gollwitzer, P. M. (2009). Goal implementation: The benefits and costs of if-then planning. In G. B. Moskowitz & H. Grant (Eds.), *The psychology of goals* (pp. 362–91). New York: Guilford Press.

Park, N., Park, M., & Peterson, C. (2010). When is the search for meaning related to life satisfaction? *Applied Psychology: Health and Well-Being, 2*(1), 1–13.

Pohlmann, K. (2001). Agency- and communion-orientation in life goals: Impact on goal pursuit strategies and psychological well-being. In P. Schmuck & K. M. Sheldon (Eds.), *Life goals and well-being: Towards a positive psychology of human striving* (pp. 68–84). Gottingen: Hogrefe & Huber.

Polivy, J., Herman, C. P., Hackett, R., & Kuleshnyk, I. (1986). The effects of self-attention and public attention on eating in restrained and unrestrained subjects. *Journal of Personality and Social Psychology, 50*(6), 1253–60.

Powers, W. T. (1973). *Behaviour: The control of perception.* Chicago, Il: Aldine.

Reeve, J., & Lee, W. (2012). Neuroscience and human motivation. In R. M. Ryan (Ed.), *The Oxford handbook of human motivation* (pp. 365–80). New York: Oxford University Press.

Riediger, M. (2007). Interference and facilitation among personal goals: Age differences and associations with well-being and behavior. In B. R. Little, K. Salmela-Aro & S. D. Phillips (Eds.), *Personal project pursuit: Goals, action, and human flourishing.* (pp. 119–43). Mahwah, NJ: Lawrence Erlbaum Associates Publishers.

Riediger, M., & Freund, A. M. (2004). Interference and Facilitation among Personal Goals: Differential Associations with Subjective Well-Being and Persistent Goal Pursuit. *Personality and Social Psychology Bulletin, 30*(12), 1511–23. doi: 10.1177/0146167204271184

Rogers, C. R. (1959). A theory of therapy, personality and interpersonal relationships as developed in the client-centered framework. In S. Koch (Ed.), *Psychology: A Study of Science* (vol. 3, pp. 184–256). New York: McGraw-Hill.

Rupani, P., Cooper, M., McArthur, K., Pybis, J., Cromarty, K., Hill, A., Levesley, R., Murdoch, J., and Turner, N. (2014). The goals of young people in school-based counselling and their achievement of these goals. *Counselling and Psychotherapy Research, 14*(4), 306–314. doi: 10.1080/14733145.2013.816758

Ryan, R. M., & Deci, E. L. (2000). Self-determination theory and the facilitation of intrinsic motivation, social development, and well-being. *American Psychologist, 55*(1), 68–78.

Ryan, R. M., & Deci, E. L. (2008). A self-determination theory approach to psychotherapy: The motivational basis for effective change. *Canadian Psychology/ Psychologie Canadienne, 49*(3), 186–93. doi: 10.1037/a0012753

Sanchez, V. C., Lewinsohn, P. M., & Larson, D. W. (1980). Assertion training: Effectiveness in the treatment of depression. *Journal of Clinical Psychology, 36*(2), 526–9.

Sartre, J.-P. (1958). *Being and Nothingness: An Essay on Phenomenological Ontology* (H. Barnes, Trans.). London: Routledge.

Schunk, D. H. (1990). Goal setting and self-efficacy during self-regulated learning. *Educational Psychologist, 25*(1), 71–86.

Sheeran, P., & Webb, T. L. (2012). From goals to action. In H. Aarts & A. J. Elliot (Eds.), *Goal-directed behavior.* New York: Psychology Press.

Sheldon, K. M., & Elliot, A. J. (1999). Goal striving, need satisfaction, and longitudinal well-being: The self-concordance model. *Journal of Personality and Social Psychology, 76*(3), 482–97. doi: 10.1037/0022-3514.76.3.482

Sheldon, K. M., & Houser-Marko, L. (2001). Self-concordance, goal attainment, and the pursuit of happiness: Can there be an upward spiral? *Journal of Personality and Social Psychology, 80*(1), 152–65. doi: 10.1037/0022-3514.80.1.152

Sheldon, K. M., & Kasser, T. (1995). Coherence and congruence: Two aspects of personality integration. *Journal of Personality and Social Psychology, 68*(3), 531–43. doi: 10.1037/0022-3514.68.3.531

Sheldon, K. M., & Kasser, T. (1998). Pursuing Personal Goals: Skills Enable Progress, but Not all Progress is Beneficial. *Personality and Social Psychology Bulletin, 24*(12), 1319–31. doi: 10.1177/01461672982412006

Spangler, W. D. (1992). Validity of questionnaire and TAT measures of need for achievement: Two meta-analyses. *Psychological bulletin, 112*(1), 140.

Steger, M. F. (2013). Experiencing meaning in life. In P. T. P. Wong (Ed.), *The human quest for meaning: Theories, research, and applications* (2nd ed., pp. 165–84). New York: Routledge.

Swift, J. K., Callahan, J. L., & Vollmer, B. M. (2011). Preferences. In J. C. Norcross (Ed.), *Psychotherapy relationships that work* (2nd ed., pp. 301–15). NY: Oxford University.

Thrash, T. M., Maruskin, L. A., & Martin, C. C. (2012). Implicit-explicit motive congruence. In R. M. Ryan (Ed.), *The Oxford handbook of human motivation* (pp. 141–156). New York: Oxford University Press.

Vos, J. (2016). Working with meaning in life in chronic or life-threatening disease: A review of its relevance and effectiveness of meaning-centred therapies. In P. Russo-Netzer, S. E. Schulenberg & A. Batthyany (Eds.), *To thrive, to cope, to understand—Meaning in positive and existential psychotherapy.* New York: Springer.

Wiese, B. S. (2007). Successful pursuit of personal goals and subjective well-being. In B. R. Little, K. Salmela-Aro & S. D. Phillips (Eds.), *Personal project pursuit: Goals, action, and human flourishing.* (pp. 301–28). Mahwah, NJ: Lawrence Erlbaum Associates Publishers.

Wiese, B. S., & Salmela-Aro, K. (2008). Goal conflict and facilitation as predictors of work-family satisfaction and engagement. [doi: DOI: 10.1016/j.jvb.2008.09.007]. *Journal of Vocational Behavior, 73*(3), 490–7.

Wilkinson, R., & Pickett, K. (2010). *The spirit level: Why equality is better for everyone.* Harmondsworth: Penguin.

Winell, M. (1987). Personal goals: The key to self-direction in adulthood. In M. E. Ford & D. H. Ford (Eds.), *Humans as self-constructing living systems: Putting the framework to work* (pp. 261–87). Hillsdale, NJ: Erlbaum.

Wolitzky, D. (2003). The theory and practice of traditional psychoanalytic treatment. In A. S. Gurman & S. B. Messer (Eds.), *Essential Psychotherapies: Theory and Practice* (2nd ed., pp. 69–106). New York: Guilford Press.

Wollburg, E., & Braukhaus, C. (2010). Goal setting in psychotherapy: The relevance of approach and avoidance goals for treatment outcome. *Psychotherapy Research, 20*(4), 488–94.

Wright, R. (2000). *Nonzero: The logic of human destiny*. NY: Vintage Books.

Chapter 4

Using goals in therapy: The perspective of people with lived experience

Amy Feltham, Kate Martin, Leanne Walker, and Lydia Harris

Drawing on the perspectives of clients who have used goals in therapy, the goals of this chapter are to explore:

◆ the importance of goal setting and the difference it can make to the experience of therapy;

◆ some of the difficulties clients can face using goals in therapy and our suggestions for therapists on how to overcome these.

Introduction

The following chapter has been written by people with lived experience of having therapy, who now work to improve healthcare services. This chapter has grown from what children, young people, and adult clients have told us about goal-setting. The majority of us are young people or young adults, but we feel the key issues are relevant to clients of all ages. It is based on our collective experience, which we hope will give you an understanding of the key themes, regardless of age, and of the importance of, issues, challenges, and tips for goal-setting from the perspective of clients with lived experience. Throughout the chapter we have included quotes from people about their views and experiences of using goals in therapy. These are from the authors' direct experience, from conversations we have had to develop this chapter, or from previous consultations we have facilitated with people to understand their experiences and advice for therapists.

As the authentic voice of people who have had therapy, this chapter aims to complement the other chapters in the book and build on what research and practice tells us about goal-setting, by exploring how goal-setting is experienced by clients. The individuals who contributed to this chapter told us about the good, the bad, and 'the ugly' in their experience of goal-setting, with the hope that it can help you use goals in therapy in a way that is as helpful for your clients as possible.

The importance of setting goals and feeling in control

We would like to begin with a case study, which looks at how goals can help us to feel in control, which we think of as one of the most important aspects of goal-setting. When we talk to people about their experiences of therapy, one of the main themes that emerges is the importance of feeling in control. This includes feeling in control over our difficulties; services received, our wider lives, information held about us, and feedback about the direction and progress of therapy. All of these aspects of control gained from the goal-setting process contribute to our ability to manage our mental health. This makes goal-setting a useful tool in therapy when done well. Leanne explains this below:

> Instead of drifting along through life getting from day to day—surviving but not living, setting goals and working on achieving them focused my life in way that nothing else had. Before working with goals in therapy, I'd had several years of counselling, and I don't wish to discredit those important years, but I had reached a standstill and I wasn't aware of how to move forward. It is then that I started CBT and I was asked 'What would you like to work to towards?'. I really struggled with this because it wasn't something I'd previously thought about, having a future 'better' than what life was then, in that moment. It was therefore important that my therapist and I spent some time discussing what I would like to be different and how I could really live and thrive—instead of just survive. From this, together (and 'together' is the operative word here), we set three goals to work towards. These goals were flexible and reshaped as we worked together and were very important in really focusing me on what I wanted to change. Each time we met we scored my progress on a scale and discussed how I could further achieve them. They were things which I had struggled with during counselling without goals but had very little idea of how to help myself and to move forward with. They helped me to see things in a different way and approach problems I had from different angles. My goals journey wasn't always easy: change is hard and, sometimes when I was struggling, change felt impossible. During such times it was very helpful to reflect back over what I had achieved. Keeping things documented was important to me to see this change. I found—when it's yourself progressing and changing—it's harder to recognize, until you look back and reflect. Then it's amazing.

The difficulties and challenges of goal-setting in therapy

The following sections will discuss some of the challenges which are often experienced when using goals, and shed light on what we, as people with lived experience, think can help to overcome these. Most of the sections begin with a quote from someone with lived experience of being in therapy. The section will then discuss the problems you might experience as a therapist and the potential solutions to these. Think of this section as a troubleshooting guide to using goals in therapy, from the people who have experienced being on the other side of the therapy room. We hope that our thoughts and experiences, combined with your experience as therapists, will help stimulate useful reflections about using goals in therapy.

However, before we do this, a word of caution from the clients we have spoken to. It is important to remember that goal-setting is not always going to be easy. In this chapter we will address some of the difficulties and solutions for professionals, but it's also important to think about how goal-setting can be difficult for us as clients. Issues such as low confidence, hopelessness, and poor previous experiences of goal-setting can make it hard for us to engage in goal-setting. The difficult but important job for you as a therapist, is to create new, manageable, and positive experiences of setting goals together with clients.

Finding a goal

YOUNG PERSON 1: It feels like I was going there to be reminded that there's something wrong with me.

GROUP: Yeah.

YOUNG PERSON 1: And also if you're in the middle of exams it can be really stressful, because it's like, well, I don't feel like you're doing anything, this is an hour I can be revising or I'm missing lessons...

YOUNG PERSON 2: I quite like missing lessons... [Group laughter]

(Young people, during a focus group exploring experiences of using goals in therapy).

In this extract, it is easy to see that the young people don't know why they're in therapy, making the process feel aimless. We know, as people who have experienced therapy, that one of the challenges you may face as a therapist is a client simply not knowing what goals to set. Many clients will not have walked through the door with pre-set goals. This may be particularly so for children and young people who may not have been involved in deciding they want or need therapy. It is important that, however old the client is, they are told that it is 'ok' not to have clear goals at the start-that they're not expected to have a 10-year plan to have goals! Reassure clients that it's ok for things to go slowly, starting with really small steps. For example, to begin with, a goal might be simply building a relationship with which the client feels comfortable, or to be able to think about the things which are important to them. These small goals can start to build understanding of goal-setting in therapy, and their confidence that they can aim for a goal and feel supported, whether it is achieved or not. This goal-setting process can in itself begin to provide them with a reason to go to therapy, creating a more fruitful relationship for everyone.

Focusing only on risk

> One of the most really weird example is: if you're in an inpatient unit, for an eating disorder or whatever—I know of people who have been on a meal plan and an exercise plan, so they have to take in a certain amount of food and they can't expend it. And some of the doctors are like, 'Oh, well you've gained weight so you must be getting better', so you're discharged and like… Well, obviously they're gonna have gained weight because you've been doing it for them, and then the minute they get out they just lose weight again. It's, like, I've had friends in that situation, in and out of the inpatients like, three or four times. Because the weight gain doesn't mean anything at all, does it, in that situation, 'cos they've not got a choice about it.
>
> (Young adult)

In this example, it is obvious that professionals are not paying attention to the whole story. From our experience of therapy, we know that when clients are at risk, it can be hard for therapists not to focus simply on keeping them safe. While managing risk is an important part of your role as a therapist, it's vital that a person's goals are thought about more holistically. Clients who have been in this situation often emphasize that only they can know what their own internal goals are, and it's important that these are explored alongside managing whatever risks there may be. So a client might have a weight gain 'goal' set by a professional but may also need to set their own goals with their therapists. These might relate to coping skills, anxiety, relationships, or a whole host of other things, and working on these can help to improve the client's quality of life and willingness to work towards a less 'risky' situation. Importantly, clients tell us that this also serves to give them a reason to do the hard work involved in therapy, and support to work towards the sort of life they want to live.

Disagreement about goals

> I don't think, like, you can—even between two people you can't say, 'This is gonna work for both of them'.
>
> (Young adult)

This quote crystallizes something that we know from our experience of therapy: sometimes the goal that makes sense to the therapist is not the one we want to set. Clearly, you and your client will not always have the same ideas about what the best goal could be. This can sometimes be seen as a difficult situation, but clients tell us that it can, in fact, be an opportunity for some really valuable therapeutic working. For this to take place, it's important to acknowledge the experience and expertise that you and your client bring, and think together about what the best way forwards might be. One way that clients have found helpful is thinking about what is important to them, the reasons the different goals are attractive, and how possible reaching the goals feels for both parties. Interestingly, this process (often referred to as a shared decision making process) can in itself be more important than the goal which is eventually set. The experience of not having your goals dismissed, being treated as of equal expertise, and negotiating an outcome can be hugely valuable.

Resistance to goal-setting

As people with experience of therapy, we know that there are a number of reasons why a client may be 'resistant' to setting a goal. This might be because of their own psychological difficulties, but might also involve other factors, such as bad experience with previous therapists. According to people with experience of *being* the resistant client, when faced with resistance to goal-setting, it might be helpful for the therapist to use a shared decision making model.

An example of this is the Open Talk model, co-developed with people with lived experience of mental health problems (Figure 4.1, Common Room, 2017). This model was developed to facilitate open conversations about decisions in therapy. Although it was primarily designed for young people's mental health services, the principles and approach apply to clients of all ages. The key aim of the model is to enable clients and therapists to have a structured decision making conversation, in which the therapist and clients can express their views, and work to reach a shared agreement.

In this model, the client and the therapist are explicit about their feelings about goal-setting, they explore the possible options around the issue, they discuss the pros and cons, and think together about what is important to them about the process of goal-setting. They also think about a way forwards where everyone's needs get taken into account. It's important to note that shared decision making does not mean doing whatever the client wants. Clients tell us that they understand that not all of their goals can be supported, and that when this is the case it's ok to say so and discuss why. What is important is the discussion, deliberation, and thinking together. The shared decision making process can still be valuable to them, showing them that they have an important and active way to be involved in their care.

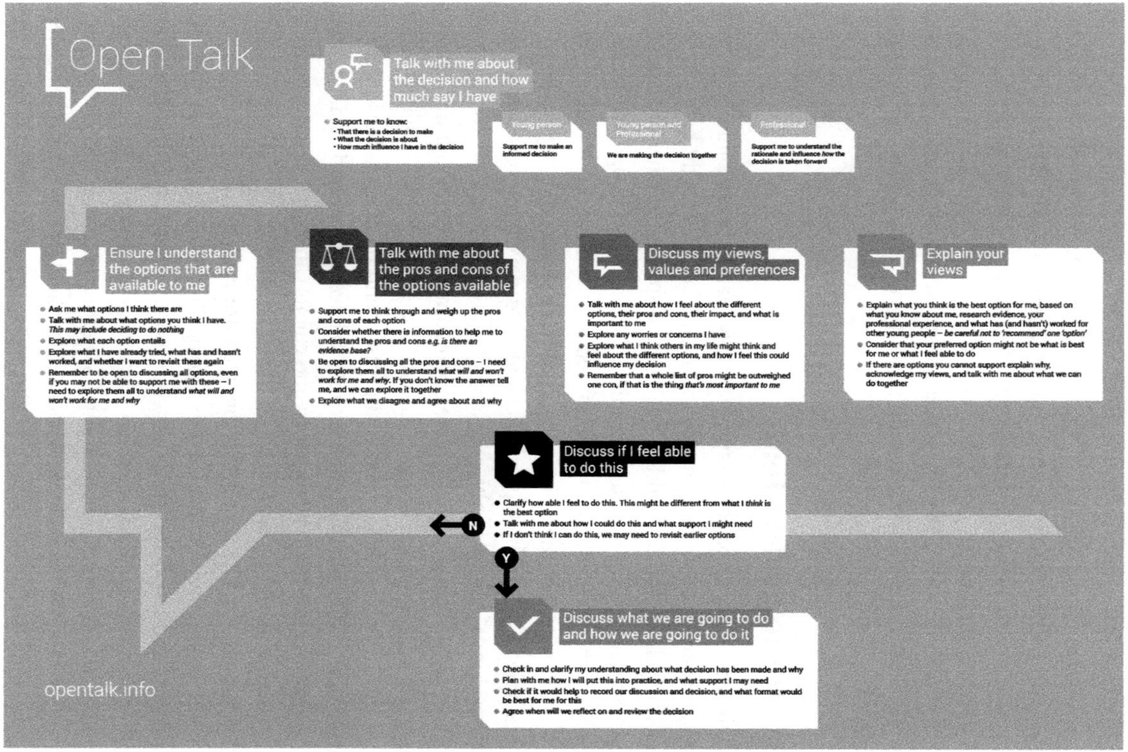

[Open Talk

Talk with me about the decision and how much I say I have
Support me to know:
- That there is a decision to make
- What the decision is about
- How much influence I have in the decision

Young person
We are making the decision together

Young person and
Professional
Support me to make an
informed decision

Professional
Support me to understand the rationale and influence how the decision is been formed

Ensure I understand the options that are available to me
- Ask me what options I think there are
- Talk with me about what options you think I have. *This may include deciding to do nothing*
- Explore what each option entails
- Explore what I have already tried, what has and hasn't worked, and whether I want to revisit these again
- Remember to be open to discussing all options, even if you may not be able to support me with these – I need to explore them all to understand what will and won't work for me and why

Talk with me about the pros and cons of the options available
- Support me to think through and weigh up the pros and cons of each option
- Consider whether there is information to help me to understand the pros and cons e.g. is there an evidence base?
- Be open to discussing all the pros and cons – I need to explore them all to understand what will and won't work for me and why. If you don't know the answer tell me, and we can explore it together
- Explore what we disagree and agree about and why

Discuss my views, values and preferences
- Talk with me about how I feel about the different options, their pros and cons, their impact, and what is important to me
- Explore any worries or concerns I have
- Explore what I think others in my life might think and feel about the different options, and how I feel this could influence my decision
- Remember that a whole list of pros might be outweighed by one con, if that is the thing that's most important to me

Explain your views
- Explain what you think is the best option for me, based on what you know about me, research evidence, your professional experience, and what has (and hasn't) worked for other young people – be careful not to 'recommend' one 'option'
- Consider that your preferred option might not be what is best for me or what I feel able to do
- If there are options you cannot support explain why, acknowledge my views, and talk with me about what we can do together

Discuss if I feel able to do this
- Clarify how able I feel to do this. This might be different from what I think is the best option
- Talk with me about how I could do this and what support I might need
- If I don't think I can do this, we may need to revisit earlier options

Discuss what we are going to do and how we are going to do it
- Check in and clarify my understanding about what decision has been made and why
- Plan with me how I will put this into practice, and what support I may need
- Check if it would help to record our discussion and decision, and what format would be best for me for this
- Agree when we will reflect on and review the decision

opentalk.info

Fig. 4.1 The Open Talk model.

Unobtainable goals

> It depends though [about what a good goal is] because if the problem is that you can't sleep, and then you can sleep, then it's fixed. But if you've got like a long-term mental health condition, the likelihood is that it's probably going to occur at some point in your life or you might always have kind of thoughts and feelings that you have to deal with. In which case you need to learn how to live with it rather than trying to get rid of it. You need to learn how to live alongside it, but it depends because something things are really short term and just get help and deal with it.
>
> (Young person)

This young person has 'hit the nail on the head' in saying that therapy cannot cure everything. For you as a therapist, it can be difficult to know how to respond to huge or unobtainable goals. While it is wonderful to hear that a client has big ambitions, you won't be able to help your client sprout wings and fly to the moon! The great thing is, we as clients know this, and mostly we think this is ok; it is not your role to get us to some huge or unobtainable milestone. What clients tell us is important is the discussion and deliberation to understand together why this may be unobtainable and to work together to agree what may be a more realistic goal. So if the client can't set that massive goal with you, what do they want to happen instead? Well, they tell us that it's important that you hear these goals and reflect in a way which doesn't leave them feeling dismissed. Sometimes clients know that they are not ready for a big goal and, again, they say that this is ok. They make clear that it is more important that the goal is right for them, rather than it being the 'gold standard' of goal-setting. It might be helpful to think about goal-setting like window cleaning. There is no point being at the top of the ladder when you're trying to clean a window on the ground floor. Similarly, it might not be fruitful to set a goal to start full-time work again when the client can barely get out of bed. It's important for the client that they know that if their goal is to start setting their alarm clock, this is ok. Clients explain that this process acknowledges their wishes and involves them in the goal-setting process.

Unsafe goals

There will always be situations where you cannot support your client's goals. From our experience, the way to start when faced with this situation is to ask yourself is 'Why can't I support this goal?'. The benefit of this is twofold. First, it prepares you to think this through with your client, explaining your logic and reasoning. Second, it encourages you to check out with yourself whether the goal really is unsafe.

When you are faced with risk situations frequently, it can be easy to become accustomed to taking away choice. For clients, this can be crushing. Therefore, asking this question can be a good way to catch yourself before telling a client you can't support a goal. For example, if a client with an eating disorder in an inpatient unit says their goal is to decide for themselves what and when they eat, this might seem like an unsafe goal. However, it may be possible to think about a safe way in which to aim for this goal and enable them to have choice about how they are supported with their eating. For example, one adult client said:

> When she started to talk to me about 'my aims' it felt stupid. I don't have any say over my life, I'm sectioned! I told her I wanted to die and she just listened and told me that she wanted something different for me, like everyone does. But once we'd been through that and she was still asking me about other 'aims' we talked about little things I want to change like trying to have a shower every day. It made me feel more like me, more like the real me was still in there somewhere. I haven't felt like that for ages.

In addition to asking yourself if and why you can't support a goal, it is important to listen to these risky goals, and keep the client talking. Sometimes, the goals a client may express at the beginning of the conversation might not be something you can agree to work on with them. However, as a client, if these are discussed rather than dismissed, the conversation might carry on. Clients tell us that it is important to think together about why they felt that was a goal they wanted to work on, what they hoped this would achieve, and explore how else you could agree to work towards this in a safer way. Although clients cannot always control their whole life, they may still have appropriate goals they want to work on. Even very small goals can give a much greater sense of control. The first conversation with a client in a risk situation may not bear fruit, but working in this way and continually opening the conversation about goals might eventually give the client the opportunity to take back some control.

Deciding how to measure goals, progress and achievements

YOUNG ADULT 1: I think you can measure some things by like, you know, numbers, though. So, like, if you say you've stopped, like, self-harming every day, to once a week; or your weight's gone up; or your bloods are better or whatever. But you have to be careful with that 'cos sometimes it can be a bit like cyclic, like, something might get better, but something else gets worse.

YOUNG ADULT 2: You do have to be kinda careful though, 'cos sometimes erm ... you might like- I know, personally, sometimes I will be self-harming less, but I'll actually be feeling a lot worse, and that's why I did it less, because I didn't have that energy to actually do it, kind of thing.

YOUNG PERSON: Like, all that stuff depends on the person. I don't think you can actually say, 'This is the way we can measure all young people's mental health and how they can get better'. Which is in some ways what they wanting to do at the moment, like they kinda want you to say, 'This is the way to measure'… I think it has to be done on person by person basis, I don't think like you can- even between two people you can't say 'This is gonna work for both of them'.

ADULT: But that's why you end up coming back. Because you haven't done it properly, you think you're better, but you're not. The outcome measure from the professionals, it seems, a lot to do with like reducing risk, so, 'This person isn't self-harming as much, so they must feel better', or 'This person's gained weight' or, 'This person is going out more', so they automatically think they must be better. And I think that's not always the case.

Here, some clients are in a focus group discussing that one of the difficulties that can easily be faced by therapists and their clients is a disagreement in the way goals should be measured. Interestingly, their experience is that this is a disagreement that can go unnoticed, as it is not always discussed when the goal is set. Therapists are often accustomed to using routine outcome measures or quantitative measurements such as frequency of self-harm to measure the progress towards a goal, whereas clients may have different ideas entirely (see Chapter 6, this volume). Their solution to stop this becoming a problem is to discuss how the goal can be measured together with the client when the goal is set. The might be a numerical or frequency measurement, might relate to keeping a diary of thoughts and feelings, or might refer to being able to do or not do things on a number of occasions. Whatever the outcome looks like, it is important that both parties have a shared understanding of this. Not doing this leaves the possibility that you are both aiming for different things.

We know from experience that recording and monitoring goals is important as it helps to keep therapy focused and enables clients to see their progress. As a client, it can feel like you are making no progress towards your goal, so recording and reflecting on the small steps along the way helps us to recognize our achievements.

YOUNG PERSON 1: I guess write positives they've achieved, and as well as what they've been suffering with … so- because, if you're just thinking about it, it can be negative in your head. But if you're writing it down, 'I did this today', and a few things you can look at because you're calm.

YOUNG PERSON 2: I think [writing goals and achievements down is] quite good …yeah. I've had diaries from when I was 12, and going back now and reading them, I think, 'Wow, I'm so much better, I'm so much healthier'.

That's quite encouraging. And even if I read them at any point, then I can gradually see myself either getting better or getting worse.

This dialogue between people who had used therapy shows how keeping a record of progress can help them to stay motivated. Sometimes, for clients, when a big goal has been set—requiring a large piece of therapeutic work—it can be difficult to see progress. There are a number of ways that this can be addressed, but recording achievements can be a great way to keep an eye on the progress of the goal. Where people have low belief in their ability to progress towards a goal this can help to encourage them along the way. And where both they and their therapist can see a lack of progress towards the goal, the recording of this may open up a conversation. This conversation might lead to a change in the way they and their therapist approach or measure the goal, or lead to a new goal completely.

Changing goals

So at the start you, like, set certain goals that you want to achieve, and they might change as you go through, and all of a sudden, if you're in a really bad place, you might not be able to see that far ahead. So you might want to keep making them and not necessarily set 10 on the first day. And once you've reached them you go, kind of thing, but I do think they need to set goals and when you reach them you can say, 'Well, that is one that's been reached, are we where we want to be or do we need to set up another one?' Also, it helps motivate you. I don't know about everyone else but when I was going through CAMHS (Child and Adolescent Mental Health Services) for about the first nine months I was like, 'Why am I even going here? I don't want to be'.

(Adult)

Here we see that, as much as we clients need goals, we also need them to be able to change as our life changes. We know from experience that this is a problem faced by a lot of therapists and their clients. When a goal is set, neither you nor your client have a crystal ball to look into the future and see whether the goal is 'right'. Often, things will go either better or worse than expected and a goal becomes less appropriate. Clients tell us that what is vital here is that the therapist and the client pick up on this and discuss it, finding a way through it together. They suggest that this might be having a temporary interim goal while things are difficult, and holding the bigger goal in mind for when the crisis has passed. It might be that the goal has been reached but the therapeutic work hasn't finished and this is a good thing to discuss with the client to allow you to agree further goals. Essentially, they say that the goal-setting process needs to be an ongoing conversation, with either party feeling able to bring up the goals to discuss and adjust again whenever they feel it is appropriate. Goal-setting can't simply be a 'set and forget' process if it is going to be successful.

Developing a shared language and understanding

Closely related to this is the issue of therapy jargon. Sometimes it can feel to clients like the therapist is speaking a different language. One young woman said:

> My [therapist] said, 'We were going to work on relationships', and I was like thinking, 'don't really understand them', because I've never had a boyfriend, and I thought that's what a relationship was, and I was like, 'I really don't get this', and she kept saying it for the first six weeks and I was like ... 'err ...' [giggles, young people in group laugh]. So I think it needs to be quite clear.... Like, use normal words.

How can we set goals together when we don't understand each other? Therapists are generally really good at avoiding jargon. However, clients say that a lot of the terms used in therapy can be jargon in disguise. Words like 'relationship' seem to have different meanings to the therapist. What is important is to check with clients about their meanings, and discuss goals in different ways to explore and check in about the meaning of the goals. Talking about the goals in a number of different ways makes sure everyone is on the same page and can access the conversation. This is not just good for the client, it also works to give the therapist a more dynamic view of the client's thoughts and feelings around the goal, which can only be a good thing therapeutically.

Different understandings of how therapy works

> We thought that it was really important for[therapists] not to be so rigid. I went to a few- I got psychotherapy and she liked to just listen rather than advise or give any support and there were instances where I'd say, 'Well, you've seen a lot more people with experiences of such-and-such, I'd like you to give me some feedback on what I should do', and she was like 'Well this is a therapy room, you're meant to talk'. And I, well, thought, 'I've run out of things to say, I want some help now, can you just, like, give me some feedback? Like some guidelines, something to help', because I was having nightmares and flashbacks and she was like, 'Well you should just talk about them'. And talking about them isn't- you know, I want some advice. Even simple advice, like, 'Do this before you go to bed', or 'Have a- have a bath'.
>
> (Adult client)

Here we see how frustrating it can be for clients when they are not getting what they expect, or even what they feel they need, from therapy, to help them reach their goals. Some clients have different ideas to their therapist about how therapy will work and this can be a big challenge when it comes to goal-setting. Some therapy styles may leave them wondering if they are really progressing towards their goals, as the therapy is not what they expected. For clients, this is a really important thing to discuss. It is important that everyone is on the same page about how you expect the client to get to their goal. Explaining the rationale behind a therapy may help them to feel that they are progressing. This discussion also enables therapists and clients to reflect on the therapeutic approach, how they are working together to think together about what is working and what may need to change.

Involvement in treatment options

As clients, we know how important it is to discuss and understand the different approaches to therapy and to reach a shared agreement with the therapist about which approach feels like the right fit. However, clients tell us that often this discussion does not happen and they feel as if a therapeutic option is being recommended rather than jointly agreed.

> Not telling you what's going to happen. Discussing it with you rather than, you know-sometimes they talk down to you a bit 'cos they might think you... don't know a lot, you're uninformed. But the thing is they need to inform you. Or they might not tell you because they think they're too above your level of intellect and they'll just ignore it and think you don't need to know that.

> (Adult client)

This therapy client makes clear that he just wanted to know what the plan was for his treatment. As people with lived experience we would go further than this, saying that clients should be actively involved in decisions about what treatment they have to help them reach their goal. Sometimes, it can be easy for a therapist not to have these discussions with their client. This often comes from a 'good' place: not wanting to overwhelm the client with information that might not make sense to them. However, clients say that an important part of the goal-setting process is that they are given the opportunity to be informed about the options regarding what the goals could be, what treatments might get them there, and how the goal might be measured. This involves them in the therapy and makes it less likely that they will be resistant to their treatment plan, as they have been involved in creating it.

Parent and child disagreeing

Children who are therapy clients also tell us that they have a specific difficulty which does not normally relate to adults. This is when their parents' goals and their own are very different. This can be a really tricky situation for the therapist to negotiate, complicated by also needing to have some input into the goals themselves. In this situation, clients say that it is really important to encourage open communication and talking about the differing goals. It might be possible to mediate, finding the common ground between different goals. Alternatively, parents tell us it might be helpful if the therapist talks to them about how their child's goals may eventually lead to their own goals (for the child) being realized.

Conclusion

We hope that this chapter has given an insight into what people with lived experience know and think about setting goals in therapy. You may have seen some themes coming up again and again in this chapter; mainly that we want to be listened to, validated, and involved in our care. This chapter is not a one-size-fits-all guide to the thoughts of therapy clients, but we hope that it can help you to think about goals from our perspective when you next discuss them with a client. Having read this chapter is an important first step in listening to people who have experience of using services: a hugely important concept as it is us you are trying to help, us who have to live with our conditions, and us who will suffer if therapeutic goals are not used well. As service users, our main wish in therapy is often to be heard, and we hope this chapter has shown that you can hear and use our goals in therapy no matter what issues might seem to get in the way.

Points for reflection

+ What do you think the main challenges are for clients when setting goals?
+ Why is goal-setting such an important part of the therapeutic process for the client?
+ What one thing could you change in your practice to make goal-setting more useful for the client?

Further reading

Common Room (2017) Open Talk decision-making model, accessed from www.opentalk. info

Law, D and Walker, L. (2015) Choosing your goals in therapy or counselling: a guide for young people. In Law, D and Jacob, J. (2015) *Goals and goals based outcomes (GBOs): some useful information.* CAMHS Press: London

Chapter 5

Goals and psychotherapy research

Georgiana Shick Tryon

The overarching goal of this chapter is to examine goals in psychotherapy as they relate to clinical outcomes by critically surveying the extant research. More specifically, the goals of this chapter are to discuss:

- the collaborative relationship between clients and psychotherapists,
- collaborative goal-setting with adult and youth clients,
- the relationship of goal consensus and progress monitoring to psychotherapy outcome,
- moderators of the goal-outcome relationship,
- implications of the research reviewed for clinical practice.

Goal-based life planning enjoys widespread popularity, as attested by an article in the *New York Times* (Parker-Pope, 2016) in which the author details how her life changed for the better when she began applying design thinking, advocated by Bernard Roth (2015), to identify obstacles in her life that kept her from reframing and achieving her goals. Indeed, most individuals have personal goals concerning what they want to achieve or avoid, and according to Emmons (2003), 'without goals, life would lack structure and purpose' (p. 106). Research results have shown that strong goal commitment, coupled with life circumstances that are favourable for goal achievement, is associated with goal attainment, which is in turn associated with increased emotional wellbeing (see Brunstein, Schultheiss, & Maier, 1999; Emmons, 2003; Freund & Riediger, 2006).

Client-therapist collaboration and psychotherapy goals

Like other individuals, psychotherapy clients have personal goals, but clients' psychotherapy goals sometimes differ from personal goals of non-clients. For instance, psychotherapy clients' goals tend to be more concrete and explicit, such as overcoming a specific fear, with definite endpoints rather than abstract motivational goals, such as becoming independent or being kind to others (Grosse Holtforth & Grawe, 2002). Jansson, Than, and Ramnerö (2015) examined the goals of adult psychotherapy clients and individuals who were not in psychotherapy. They found that clients tended to have more goals 'related to depressive symptoms, substance abuse, and coping with somatic problems ... compared to the non-client group' (p. 187), and clients also endorsed fewer interpersonal goals and goals related to past, present, and future events than did non-clients. Clients were more likely to believe that they were further from reaching their goals than were non-clients. These results indicate that clients choose goals that concentrate on their symptoms/problems, and perhaps because they have been struggling with their problems for some time, they do not see these goals as being resolved in the near future.

Relative to non-clients, psychotherapy clients tend to have more avoidance goals concerning situations or emotions that they want to avoid (Grosse Holtforth, Bents, Mauler, & Grawe, 2006). Several studies have associated clients' avoidance goals, such as not stressing about work, not being afraid, and not being self-destructive, with greater symptomatology (Dickson & MacLeod, 2004; Elliot & Church, 2002; Grosse Holtforth, Grawe, Egger, & Berking, 2005). But what is perhaps most unique about psychotherapy goals is that their formulation generally results from a collaboration between client and psychotherapist, and there is research evidence that this collaboration is related to client outcomes.

Collaboration in psychotherapy

It is difficult to imagine how clients and psychotherapists would find consensus on psychotherapy goals and how to reach them without collaborating with each other. Collaboration is an active process whereby client and therapist engage in a discussion about what goals to work toward in psychotherapy and how to work toward them. Clients generally come to therapy with problems that have made their lives difficult and that they have tried, but failed, to solve. Therapists bring skills gleaned from their training and experience that can be used to help clients address their problems successfully. Collaboration between therapist and client entails a mutual discussion that begins with the therapist asking the client what brought him or her to therapy and what the client hopes to achieve in therapy. Some clients have concise, specific goals, such as to be able to fly on a plane without experiencing anxiety. Others have more general goals that need to be clarified, such as a desire to be happier. To facilitate a clearly defined goal, the therapist must ask for specific examples of what 'being happier' would entail.

Collaboration is the process of client reflection on and communication of what he or she would like from psychotherapy coupled with the therapist listening to and clarifying what the client wants to achieve and suggesting how the therapy process will proceed to enable goal achievement. The collaborative process continues throughout therapy as goals and the methods to achieve them are modified depending on what occurs. In short, client-therapist collaboration to achieve a consensus on psychotherapy goals appears necessary; otherwise, therapy will have no agreed direction.

That said, there is no consensus in the research literature about what constitutes a good collaboration or how to measure it. Bachelor, Laverdière, Gamache, and Bordeleau (2007) asked adult clients to describe their psychotherapy collaboration experiences and found that clients' perceptions of what constitutes a good collaboration varied according to the emphasis they placed on their own contribution to the work of psychotherapy, which includes goal formulation, on a continuum from very active to very therapist-dependent. Although all clients emphasized psychotherapists' active involvement in the psychotherapy process, the greater the emphasis that clients placed on their own responsibility for productive therapy work, the less responsibility they placed on their therapists.

In our meta-analysis (i.e. statistical integration of the results of several independent studies), Greta Winograd and I (Tryon & Winograd, 2011) examined the collaboration-outcome relationship in 19 studies with a total of 2260 adult psychotherapy clients that used a variety of measures of collaboration, including instruments looking at clients' role involvement and cooperation as well as client and therapist mutual involvement in the psychotherapy process. Clients' collaboration was often assessed by the quantity and quality of homework completed, by clients' ratings of their commitment to therapy, and by therapists' ratings of how involved the clients were in activities such as self-disclosure and working productively with therapists' suggestions. Therapists' collaboration was assessed by clients' ratings of therapists' understanding and helpfulness. The meta-analysis yielded an average correlation of .33 between client-therapist collaboration and psychotherapy outcome. A correlation of this magnitude represents a medium effect, which Cohen (1992) describes as 'an effect likely to be visible to the naked eye of a careful observer' (p. 156). Thus, one would expect that an individual who observes a course of psychotherapy would be able to see from the behaviour of client and psychotherapist that there is a relationship between the degree of their collaboration and the outcome the client achieves, such that greater collaboration is associated with a better outcome.

Collaboration in psychotherapy with children and adolescents usually includes the youth, his or her parents/caregivers, and the psychotherapist, and is further complicated by younger children possibly not having sufficient cognitive development to understand the process whereby psychotherapy goals and the tasks to achieve them are developed (Shirk, Karver, & Brown, 2011). Similar to adult psychotherapy, there is no consensus on how to measure collaboration in psychotherapy with youths. Results of a meta-analysis of 49 studies by Karver, Handelsman, Fields, and Bickman (2006), however, provide some indication of the collaboration-outcome relationship in child and adolescent psychotherapy by investigating the relationship between psychotherapy outcome and parent and youth participation in therapy, which they defined as 'the client's (parent or youth) effort, involvement, collaboration, cooperation, and engagement in therapy or therapy homework tasks' (p. 53). The effect size (i.e. average correlation) for youth participation-outcome was .27 (a medium effect), and for parent participation-outcome was .26[1] (also a medium effect). Thus, there is reason to believe that collaboration assessed by participation of both parent and youth clients with their psychotherapists is related to better child/adolescent psychotherapy outcomes.

Collaborative goal-setting

Several authors emphasize the importance of client-psychotherapist collaborative goal-setting in psychotherapy (Cooper & McLeod, 2007; Duncan & Reese, 2015; DeFife & Hilsenroth, 2011; Ryan & Deci, 2008), and stress that the inclusion of clients in goal-setting enhances their motivation to participate in treatment (Ryan, Lynch, Vansteenkiste, & Deci, 2011). Not all clients are motivated to engage fully in the psychotherapy process. Some begin treatment with scepticism or hopelessness about its effectiveness. Others come to therapy because of outside pressures rather than of their own volition. When clients are not fully motivated, therapy may not be effective, and clients may not even stay in therapy. Collaboration engages the client to participate actively in choosing the goals of psychotherapy, which mobilizes the client to work toward what he or she has chosen, thereby increasing the client's motivation for treatment. Goldman, Hilsenroth, Owen, and Gold (2013) found that when therapists collaborate with their clients in setting therapy goals and defining the course of treatment, clients are likely to agree with and have confidence in the treatment process. Research results indicate, however, that

---

[1] This effect size does not include results of one study of frequent reporting of abuse that Karver et al. (2006) indicated represented a treatment that was atypical.

achieving collaborative goal consensus is not an easy task, nor is it always successful.

With adults

Although some adult clients and psychotherapists readily come to agreement on treatment goals, others do not. For example, Swift and Callahan (2009) asked clients and clinical psychology trainee psychotherapists to specify the two most important goals that they were working on after the third therapy session. Client and psychotherapist identified the same two goals only 31.1% of the time; they agreed on one of the two goals 56.3% of the time; and they did not match on either target goal 12.6% of the time. Lest readers think that the lack of goal agreement in this study is solely the result of psychotherapist inexperience, results of a study by Zane et al. (2005) indicated that experienced psychotherapists sometimes do not agree with their clients about treatment goals. In this study, client-psychotherapist goal match predicted client-rated session depth and smoothness as well as session positivity. In other words, client-therapist goal consensus is associated with deeper, more meaningful, smoother, and more positive psychotherapy sessions. If, on the other hand, there is disagreement between client and therapist about goals, they will find it difficult to work toward an agreeable session outcome, because there is doubt on the part of the client, the therapist, or both about the direction that the session should take. So, for one or both members of the therapeutic dyad, the session will seem superficial and without much value. Because client and therapist are 'not on the same page', the session will not go smoothly. The client may argue with the therapist or contribute little information; the therapist may express frustration with the client's behaviour. Neither will evaluate the session positively, and one can imagine that if goal consensus is not achieved, future sessions, if they occur at all, will also have little positive effect.

Results of one study suggest that adult clients sometimes place more emphasis on collaborative goal consensus than do their psychotherapists. Bachelor (2013) examined clients' and psychotherapists' perceptions of their work together. Both emphasized a collaborative working relationship, but only clients stressed the importance of non-disagreement on goals. Notably, it was clients' view of the relationship that better predicted psychotherapy outcome. Bachelor indicated that the results suggest that therapists should not conclude that clients share their views about their work together, but should regularly check with clients to get their feedback on how therapy is progressing. 'Therapists should ensure that goals and therapeutic tasks are discussed together and mutually determined and remain vigilant for signs of tension in the relationship that could reflect a perceived lack of shared views, adjusting their responses accordingly' (Bachelor, p. 133).

Several authors (Cooper & McLeod, 2007; Michalak & Grosse Holtforth, 2006) have emphasized the importance of continued collaborative goal review throughout psychotherapy. Evidence suggests that when psychotherapists change goals during the course of psychotherapy without agreement of their clients, treatment outcome is adversely affected (Schulte-Bahrenberg & Schulte, 1993).

To assist practitioners to foster better collaboration with clients, researchers have developed procedures that facilitate systematic client feedback on psychotherapy goals and the tasks to achieve them throughout the process of psychotherapy (Duncan, 2012; Duncan & Reese, 2015; Goldman et al., 2013; Lambert, 2010; Lambert & Shimokawa, 2011). A review of 32 studies (Gondek, Edbrooke-Childs, Fink, Deighton, & Wolpert, 2016) that used feedback found that, relative to no-feedback or other experimental conditions, treatments that incorporated feedback had better outcomes on at least one measure and were particularly effective when feedback was provided to both clients and psychotherapists.

Another review by Davidson, Perry, and Bell (2015), however, indicated that many feedback studies were done with mildly disturbed college student clients, and that results may be less positive when clients have more severe disturbances. In that vein, a recent study by Lucock and colleagues (2015) with clients from the UK National Health Service (NHS) found that clients treated at two UK NHS centres that use patient monitoring and feedback improved with treatment, but they did not show significantly greater improvement than did clients at another UK NHS site that did not use feedback. Thus, feedback to clients about treatment progress (i.e. progress toward their goals) may be more helpful for clients with milder disturbances than for clients with more severe problems.

With youths

Youth, particularly children, usually do not decide to enter therapy on their own. Many do not believe that their behaviour presents a problem, nor do they necessarily know why parents/caregivers bring them for help. A few days after intake, Yeh and Weisz (2001) asked 381 parents and their children to list the children's target problems independently. Almost two-thirds (63%) of parent-child pairs failed to agree on even one problem. When the authors grouped parents' and children's responses into broader categories, over a third of the parent-child responses did not fall into the same broad problem area, such as withdrawn or aggressive behaviour.

Parents may have goals for youth with problems that are not shared by their children or, for that matter, by their psychotherapists. Thus, it is not surprising that in a study of 315 children, parents, and psychotherapists, Hawley and Weisz (2003) found that only 23.2% of the members of the triad agreed on any target problem, or put another way, 'when asked to report the main problems in need of treatment, 76.8% did not agree on a single target problem' (p. 65). Garland, Lewczyk-Boxmeyer, Gabayan, and Hawley (2004) reported similar findings for adolescent clients.

In a more recent study, Stafford, Hutchby, Karim, and O'Reilly (2016) found that half of their sample of clinicians did not bother to ask child clients why they came for psychotherapy and what they expected to occur. This does not seem a good way to initiate goal collaboration. In contrast, results of another study (Diamond, Liddle, Hogue, & Dakof, 1999) found that psychotherapist behaviours associated with good treatment alliances involved telling adolescents that their stated problems are important, asking what concerns adolescents want help with, and indicating that they will advocate for the youth. In cases with poorer client-therapist relationships, psychotherapists did not engage in these collaborative goal-setting behaviours. Others (Coatsworth, Santisteban, McBride, & Szapocznik, 2001; Faw, Hogue, Johnson, Diamond, & Liddle, 2005) have reported the effectiveness of psychotherapists' engagement in similar behaviours with youth and family members to negotiate goals that include each family member's concerns.

Garland, Hawley, Brookman-Frazee, and Hurlburt (2008) reviewed the manuals of eight treatments for children with disruptive disorders and found that collaborative agreement on psychotherapy goals, which includes periodic reviews of goals and progress toward them, is a core element of evidence-based treatments. Collaboration, described as 'therapist building togetherness with the child client', associated with goal-setting has also been related to a positive child-therapist working relationship using manualized treatment for anxiety disorders (Creed & Kendall, 2005, p. 503). In the UK, shared decision making (SDM) has been implemented in Child and Adolescent Mental Health Services (CAMHS) in recognition of the importance of including children and adolescents as well as parents/caregivers and other stakeholders in continuing collaborative goal-setting and treatment evaluations (Abrines-Jaume et al., 2016; Hoong, Heathfield, Fitzpatrick, & Benson, 2014; Law & Jacob, 2013; Law & Wolpert, 2014).

Goals and psychotherapy outcomes

One of the main reasons to engage in collaborative goal-setting is to establish an endpoint for clients and their psychotherapists to work toward. Hopefully, during psychotherapy, the goals will be reached, and clients will be better off as a result.

Goal consensus and goal progress monitoring and their relationships with outcome in adult clients

Greta Winograd and I (Tryon & Winograd, 2011) examined the relationship of client-psychotherapist goal consensus and psychotherapy outcome via a meta-analysis of 15 studies with a total of 1302 adult clients. Goal consensus measures included assessments of client-psychotherapist goal agreement, client-psychotherapist congruence on the origin of clients' problems, and client-therapist agreement on the expectations of psychotherapy. Some of the goal measures were subscales of working alliance measures, such as the Working Alliance Inventory (WAI; Horvath & Greenberg, 1989) and the California Psychotherapy Alliance Scale (CALPAS; Marmar, Horowitz, Weiss, & Marziali, 1989), whereas others were constructed by the authors of each particular study. Psychotherapy outcome was assessed by examining post-therapy improvement on several standard measures of symptoms (most studies used more than one outcome measures), such as the Beck Depression Inventory (BDI), the Brief Symptoms Inventory (BSI), the Symptom Checklist-90 (SCL-90), the Hamilton Rating Scale for Depression (HAMD), and Yale-Brown Obsessive Compulsive Scale (Y-BOCS), as well as by treatment dropout, behavioural avoidance tests, and therapist and client ratings of improvement. The majority of outcome ratings were made by clients.

We found a positive, medium effect size of .34 between client-therapist goal consensus and psychotherapy outcome. This finding suggests that client-psychotherapist agreement on goals is related to better client outcomes. Readers should note that the studies in the meta-analysis usually measured goal consensus at just one point during psychotherapy, and usually this assessment happened early in treatment. This suggests that practitioners who establish goal consensus with their clients early in psychotherapy are likely to achieve better outcomes.

Another meta-analysis examined the relationship between goal progress monitoring and outcome in 138 studies with a total of 19 951 adult participants (Harkin et al., 2016). All of the studies randomly assigned adults to a treatment that monitored goal progress or to a control condition (i.e. a comparative treatment that may have included some monitoring, but of a different type or to a lesser degree or to a no-treatment control). The studies monitored a variety of outcomes including mood, depressive symptoms, physical activity, medication compliance, weight, diet, and time management. Harkin and colleagues found an average correlation of .20[2] between goal monitoring and outcome, which represents a small

---

[2] Harkin et al. (2016) reported this effect size as $d = .40$. To ensure consistent reporting of effect sizes, I converted this effect and the other effects from articles reported in this chapter to correlations (r) using software on the Psychometrica webpage at http://www.psychometrica.de/effect_size.html.

to medium effect size. This result suggests that treatments that include goal monitoring are associated with better outcomes for a variety of concerns.

Taken together, the results of these two meta-analytic publications (Harkin et al., 2016; Tryon & Winograd, 2011) suggest that therapists who work collaboratively with clients at the beginning of treatment to determine why they came to psychotherapy and what they want to achieve and then monitor progress toward these agreed goals are more likely to have better outcomes than therapists who do not engage in these activities.

Moderators of the goal-outcome relationship

The results of the meta-analyses reported above indicate that goals and outcomes are positively related, but that the relationship between psychotherapy goals and outcomes is not always the same. Other variables, called moderators, can influence the strength of the relationship between goals and outcomes. In the Harkin et al. (2016) study, one moderator of the goal monitoring-outcome relationship was problem type. Thus, the relationship between goal monitoring and outcome represented a medium effect of .31 when the clients' problems dealt with depression, and a small effect of .15 when the clients' problems dealt with dieting. So, if you observed psychotherapy for each of these two types of problems, you might notice more improvement when clients had monitored goals related to depression than when clients had monitored goals related to weight loss. In similar manner, if a client's goal was to increase his or her physical activity (effect size $r = .28$), monitoring might be associated with greater gains than if a client's goal was to follow a diet ($r = .11$).

The relationship between goal monitoring and outcome was also stronger when participants' monitoring was physically recorded by clients on a form or in a diary ($r = .21$, a small to medium effect) and publicized (monitored in public, such as weighing oneself in front of another, or sharing with others in written form) ($r = .26$, a small to medium effect) than when the monitoring was not recorded ($r = .14$, a small effect) and the information was kept private ($r = .09$, a small effect). When clients make a record of their goal progress, they can refer to it both with their therapists and between sessions. Physical recordings that clients make and retain can prompt clients to continue toward their goals by allowing concrete examination of where they have started, where they are now, and how far they have to go to achieve their goals. When clients share self-monitoring records with therapists, and perhaps with others as well, they may feel a greater commitment to progress toward goals because of a belief that therapists will hold them accountable. Thus, goals that are monitored by clients themselves, recorded, and publicized are associated with better outcomes than are goals that are monitored but not recorded and not publicized.

Other types of goals have also been found to moderate, or change the strength of, the goal-outcome relationship. For instance, avoidance goals (i.e. things that clients are motivated to avoid, see Chapter 3, this volume) have been associated with greater client symptomatology (e.g. clients who have more avoidance goals tend to have greater psychopathology), and studies also show that they are related to more negative psychotherapy outcomes. For example, a client may have an avoidance goal to stop being so self-critical. To achieve this goal, the client may criticize herself whenever she finds herself being self-critical. This behaviour might lead to a feeling of hopelessness about ever being able to reach her goal and an increase in her cycle of self-criticism. If, on the other hand, the client frames her goal as being kinder to herself (an approach goal), she will look for ways to reward herself for the behaviours she likes. Readers should note that clients' avoidance goals can often be reframed as approach goals that are more attainable than avoidance goals but still address the clients' problems, such as in the example just presented.

Elliot and Church (2002) found that adult clients who had more avoidance goals were less satisfied with their psychotherapists, and tended to have smaller increases in subjective wellbeing over the course of psychotherapy than did clients who had fewer avoidance goals. Avoidance goals were also negatively related to perceived problem improvement at termination. Grosse Holtforth et al. (2005) found that avoidance goal motivation of 76 outpatients decreased over the course of psychotherapy. The decline in intensity of all types of avoidance goals combined related to improvement in interpersonal problems and optimism, as well as attainment of other treatment goals. Declines in avoidance goals associated with vulnerability (e.g. to stop being emotionally overwhelmed, to stop showing weakness) were more strongly related to interpersonal, symptom, and optimism improvement than were other avoidance goals, such as to stop being lonely or embarrassed.

In a further study, Grosse Holtforth et al. (2006) examined interpersonal problems of 284 clinic clients relative to their approach and avoidance goals. They found that both avoidance goals and interpersonal distress were negatively related to achievement of approach goals. Moreover, interpersonal distress moderated (i.e. changed the strength of) the relationship of avoidance goals to achievement of approach goals such that lesser interpersonal distress was associated with a less intense negative relationship between avoidance goals and approach goal attainment. Thus, clients with fewer interpersonal concerns were more likely to achieve therapy approach goals even though they had some avoidance goals than were clients with more interpersonal concerns. Another study (Wollburg & Braukhaus, 2010) found that, although having avoidance goals did not affect goal attainment, clients who had avoidance goals achieved less symptom improvement than did clients who had only approach goals.

Intrinsic goals (i.e. goals that are rewarding in themselves, such as learning something for the pleasure gained from that knowledge, see Chapter 3, this volume) are also associated with better psychological outcomes (i.e. stronger goal-outcome relationships) than are extrinsic goals (i.e. goals that are external to the client, such as learning something because it is required to obtain a grade or satisfy some other requirement). Michalak, Klapphack, and Kosfelder (2004) found that clients who had more intrinsically oriented personal goals and who were more optimistic about attaining those goals had better session outcomes and less psychopathology (i.e. the study showed that people who set intrinsic goals are less disturbed) than did clients whose goals were more extrinsic and who were less optimistic about attaining them. The intrinsic goals in this study were general life goals, such as being a good person, husband, or parent, and did not necessarily focus on symptom relief. In another study (Ryan, Plant, & O'Malley, 1995), 109 adults with alcohol problems who were in treatment because of external pressures from family or legal authorities (i.e. had extrinsically motivated goals) were less involved in their treatment and more likely to drop out than were clients who chose to participate on their own (i.e. had intrinsically motivated goals).

Other types of goals besides approach/avoidance goals and intrinsic/extrinsic goals also may moderate the goal-outcome relationship. Using the Bern Inventory of Treatment Goals (BIT-T; Grosse Holtforth & Grawe, 2002), Berking, Grosse Holtforth, Jacobi, and Kröner-Herwig (2005) examined the treatment goals of 2770 adult inpatients to determine if some types of goals are easier to attain (i.e. yielded better goal-outcome relationships) than others. They found that, of the five general BIT-T goal categories, wellbeing-related goals (such as learning to relax, increasing calmness, improving leisure activities) were most often attained, followed in order by interpersonal, personal growth, symptom-related, and existential goals (such as coming to terms with one's past or reflecting on the future). The most attained specific goals dealt with panic attacks and self-acceptance, and the least attained specific goals dealt with chronic pain and sleep problems. The authors suggested that psychotherapists motivate clients to choose attainable goals based on the results of their research by explaining that the goals that the clients want may be more difficult to attain than a similar, but related, goal. Berking et al. provide the following example: 'If a patient wants to work on a sleep disorder problem, the goal 'to learn how to cope with my sleeping problems' is more appropriate than the goal 'to get rid of my sleeping problems'" (p. 322). The authors stress, however, that clients must be fully accepting of any reformulation of goals; otherwise, it may be best to stick with the original goal formulation because clients may not have the motivation to do otherwise.

Goals as psychotherapy outcomes

Most studies of goals use measures of general functioning or standardized symptom inventories to assess psychotherapy outcomes. But, because clients and their psychotherapists have treatment goals, it makes sense to assess those goals specifically at termination. Thus, degree of goal attainment can be used as a measure of outcome with both adults and children (see Chapter 6, this volume). Shefler, Canetti, and Wiseman (2001) used trained judges to construct individual Goal Attainment Scales (GAS) for 33 clients in short-term psychotherapy based on intake transcripts. The scales addressed five content areas (symptoms, self-esteem, romantic relations, same-sex friendships, and work performance). Termination and six-month follow-up GAS scores were significantly related to scores on standard measures of outcome such as the Brief Symptom Inventory and the Rosenberg Self-Esteem Scale. Thus, results supported the use of GAS as a measure of outcome.

Grosse Holtforth, Reubi, Ruckstuhl, Berking, and Grawe (2004) asked 675 inpatients to list three individual treatment goals at their admission to hospital. At the end of hospitalization, patients rated their goals on a 6-point scale where higher numbers indicated greater goal attainment. The ratings showed substantial improvement across most goal categories, especially those that tapped symptoms and wellness.

In a study by Proctor and Hargate (2013), 477 outpatient adults completed the Goal Attainment Form (GAF), which asked them to identify at the beginning of psychotherapy as many as four difficulties they hoped to address and to rate the degree to which they were helped with the difficulties at termination from psychotherapy. Clients also completed the Clinical Outcomes for Routine Evaluation-Outcome Measure (CORE-OM) at both the beginning and the end of psychotherapy. In the UK, the CORE-OM is a widely used and researched measure of psychological distress (Barkham, Mellor-Clark, Connell, & Cahill, 2006). The relationship between clients' GAF and change in CORE-OM scores at termination was a -.27 (a medium effect), which suggests that improvements in clients' goal concerns were associated with less psychological distress. The authors concluded that this correlation 'suggests that the GAF is measuring something different from the CORE-OM and justifies its use as a separate measure, perhaps providing a clearer client perspective on what they consider to be improvement and how much this is due to therapy' (p. 240).

The goal-outcome relationship with child and adolescent clients

Unfortunately, there are no large meta-analyses of research on the goal-outcome relationship with youth[3], but that does not mean that goals are unimportant in psychotherapy with youth. Indeed, one study (Grossoehme & Gerbetz, 2004) found that, at discharge from hospital for mental health problems, former adolescent inpatients (aged 11-18) rated goal-setting work along with peer goal contacts as one of their most meaningful experiences.

Goal consensus and outcome

Similar to findings with adult clients, youth goal consensus with psychotherapists appears related to outcome. Auerbach, May, Stevens, and Kiesler (2008) studied 39 inner-city adolescent substance-abusing clients who received three months of intensive treatment. They and their psychotherapists rated their goal consensus on the goal subscale of the WAI during the second week of treatment. The relationship between client-therapist goal consensus represented only a very small effect ($r = .07$); furthermore, the difference between client-therapist goal ratings predicted client illegal activities at outcome ($r = .38$, a medium effect), indicating that larger disparities in goal consensus were related to poorer adolescent outcomes.

Pereira, Lock, and Oggins (2006) examined goal consensus ratings of 41 adolescent girls and parents with their psychotherapists during manualized family-based therapy to empower parents to take responsibility for changing adolescents' eating behaviours and gradually return responsibility of eating to the adolescents themselves. Three clinical psychology graduate students rated adolescent-therapist and parent-therapist goal consensus early (after approximately one to two months) and later (after approximately eight to nine months) in treatment using the goal subscale of the observer form of the WAI. Adolescent weight gain was associated with greater early therapy client-therapist goal consensus ($r = .33$, medium effect). Thus, as with adult clients, it seems important to establish client-therapist goal consensus to achieve better therapy outcomes.

Goals and treatment continuation

Treatment continuation, or lack thereof, is akin to psychotherapy outcome because clients are more likely to have better outcomes if they remain until

---

[3] Although there have been meta-analyses (McLeod, 2011; Shirk, Karver, & Brown, 2011) of youth-therapist working alliance-outcome studies that included measures of the working alliance such as the WAI, which has a goal subscale, the studies did not examine subscales in their alliance-outcome analyses.

psychotherapy is completed. Citing studies that showed that approximately half of families terminate psychotherapy prematurely, Brookman-Frazee, Haine, Gabayan, and Garland (2008) examined the goal agreement of 169 youth (aged 11–18), their parents/caregivers, and their therapists in community-based psychotherapy. When parents and youth agreed on at least one goal at intake, the youth attended greater numbers of sessions than when there was no parent-child goal consensus. Youth-therapist consensus and parent-therapist consensus on at least one goal at intake was unrelated to number of sessions attended. This result suggested that therapists should facilitate initial parent-youth goal consensus to keep youth in treatment longer.

Others have found that parent/caregiver goal consensus is important in youth treatment continuation; however, the person with whom parents have consensus often differs. For example, Pereira et al. (2006) found that early parent-therapist goal consensus was significantly related to continuation in therapy ($r = .35$, medium effect) for adolescents with eating disorders. Adolescent-therapist goal consensus, although in the positive direction, was not significantly related to continuation in psychotherapy ($r = .21$, small to medium effect).

Finally, others have emphasized the importance of goal consensus among youth, parents, and psychotherapists for psychotherapy continuation without providing consensus data for participant pairings. For example, Coatsworth et al. (2001) cited low rates of engagement (i.e. client return for psychotherapy after intake assessment) and treatment retention of families who seek help for youth behaviour problems. They compared engagement and retention of families who received Brief Strategic Family Therapy (BSFT) and those who received community-based treatment as usual. BSFT emphasizes collaborative agreement on treatment goals among therapy participants. Families who participated in this goal-directed psychotherapy were more likely to engage in treatment initially ($r = .22$, small to medium effect) and to stay in treatment ($r = .30$, medium effect) than were families receiving treatment as usual.

Goals as outcome

Similar to studies with adult clients, researchers have used idiographic (individually customized) measures to examine goal achievement in psychotherapy with youth (see Chapter 6, this volume). Weisz et al. (2011) incorporated the pretreatment perspectives of 178 children (aged 7-13) and their parents who independently identified three top problems and rated their severity weekly on a 10-point scale. Youth and caregivers also completed standardized outcome measurements. The top problems information complemented the results obtained from the standardized measures by providing very specific information about problems that were high-priority treatment targets for youth and their parents that were not covered by items in standardized narrow band clinical scales. 'For example, for 41% of caregivers and 79% of youths, the identified top problems did not correspond to any items of any narrowband scales in the clinical range' (p. 369). Top problems scores were reliable and showed sensitivity to change.

Several studies conducted in the UK have used idiographic Goal Based Outcome (GBO) assessments (Law & Wolpert, 2014) to both guide and evaluate psychotherapy with youth. Wolpert et al. (2012) used GBO wherein therapist, youth, and caregiver identified collaboratively up to three goals within the first three sessions that were rated on a 10-point scale, where higher values mean greater goal achievement, at the beginning and end of treatment. Caregivers and youth also completed the standardized measure Strengths and Difficulties Questionnaire (SDQ) at the first session and after six months. Practitioners completed two standardized measures: after first meeting and after six months. GBO scores showed statistically significant improvement in goal achievement at the end relative to the beginning of treatment ($r = .69$, a large effect). GBO pre-post difference scores were related to pre-post scores on standardized measures completed by both caregivers and psychotherapists with most correlations representing medium effects (range of $r = .26$ to $r = .39$). Thus, the authors concluded that idiographic collaboratively identified goal attainment can be used in conjunction with more standardized measures to assess youth psychotherapy outcome.

In another study, Edbrooke-Childs, Jacob, Law, Deighton, and Wolpert (2015) compared data, collected over the course of several years, using SDQ and GBO scores from treatment cases involving 137 children, aged 0–18, that were completed early in and after four to six months of treatment and compared with psychotherapists' ratings of youths' global functioning. GBO scores showed greater change at outcome ($r = .76$, large effect) than did the SDQ ratings of change in psychosocial difficulties ($r = .22$, small to medium effect) and impact on daily life ($r = .41$, medium to large effect), and importantly, GBO scores were uniquely associated with psychotherapist-reported change in functioning over treatment ($r = .45$, medium to large effect). A meta-analysis using combined GBO data from three randomized controlled trials of humanistic school-based counselling for distressed youth (Cooper et al., 2010; McArthur, Cooper, & Berdondini, 2013; Pybis et al., 2014) found medium effects for improvements in goal outcomes at six and 12 weeks of treatment ($r = .31$, $r = 30$, respectively). Results support the importance of including goals in outcome evaluations.

Conclusions and causality

The research reviewed in this chapter suggests that client-psychotherapist collaboration and goal consensus is related to better psychotherapy outcomes for both adult and youth clients. For adults, the goal-outcome relationship is moderated by goal type, problem type, and recording of goal monitoring. Child goal-outcome research has not yet yielded moderators. Further, collaborative goal-based treatments with both youth and adult clients are associated with better outcomes as measured by both standardized and idiographic assessments.

Does this mean that collaborative goal-setting causes better outcomes? Causality is difficult to establish because relationships do not always mean that one thing causes another; for example, both could be caused by other, unmeasured variables. Although newer studies of goal consensus and outcome include other variables related to outcome in addition to goal consensus, it is impossible to include, or probably even surmise, all the variables that are important to the goal consensus-psychotherapy outcome.

Our methods of assessment are less than perfect, and unreliable measures lack validity. Thus, studies that use unreliable measures do not add to causal conclusions concerning psychotherapy goals and outcomes. Some studies have assessed client-psychotherapist goal consensus using idiographic instruments constructed by the authors that occasionally consist of just one item. It is not possible to judge the reliability of single-item ratings of a construct such as goal consensus. Other measures, however, such as the goal subscale of the WAI and its shorter version (the WAI-S, Tracey & Kokotovic, 1989), have demonstrated good to excellent reliability in numerous studies and can be used in practice as well as research. Readers of studies that employ standard measures such as the WAI can be more certain of the validity of the conclusions drawn by their authors.

Samples in published studies may consist of clients who are different in important ways from clients with whom readers practice. For instance, studies using feedback have often been done with college students who may not demonstrate the same level of psychopathology as clients in outpatient clinics or hospitals, and the level of client pathology may relate to the results achieved. Thus, results that apply to one type of client may not apply to others.

Much of the research on psychotherapy goals relies on correlational statistics, which generally do not support causative conclusions. Newer studies that use more sophisticated designs and statistics, such as structural equation modelling, permit some assurance of a causal relationship. Meta-analyses, such as those cited in this chapter, that aggregate data from several studies across many clients and psychotherapists allow for more definitive conclusions. In their inferences based on meta-analyses of several psychotherapy relationship variables, Norcross and Wampold (2011) indicated that goal consensus and collaboration between adults and their psychotherapists are 'probably effective' (p. 99) in improving client outcomes, but more studies are needed before these elements are deemed 'demonstrably effective'. Indeed, more goal-outcome research with both youth and adult clients is needed to clarify the goal-outcome relationship.

Summary and suggestions for practitioners

Suggestions for practitioners are presented throughout this chapter and summarized here. The research literature reviewed indicates that practitioners who want to achieve better client outcomes should:

◆ ask clients at intake why they come to psychotherapy and what they want to achieve,

◆ collaborate with clients to determine specific treatment goals and ways to achieve them,

◆ determine that clients are fully committed to achieving their goals,

◆ include parent/caregiver and youth in goal-setting, making sure to satisfy the wishes of both,

◆ direct clients to set more approach than avoidance goals,

◆ direct clients to set goals that are intrinsic rather than extrinsic,

◆ direct clients to set goals that are more easily attained,

◆ physically record and regularly review goals and goal progress with clients.

Points for reflection

◆ How do you think the literature reviewed in this chapter will inform your clinical practice?

◆ Imagine you have an adolescent client and parents who disagree with each other about treatment goals. How would you address this issue given the literature reviewed in this chapter?

◆ Think of some client goals that may be difficult to attain. How would you address them with the client given the research presented in this chapter?

Further reading

Karoly, P., & Anderson, C. W. (2000). The long and short psychological change: Toward a goal-centered understanding of treatment durability and adaptive success. In C. R.

Snyder & R. E. Ingram (Eds.), *Handbook of psychological change* (pp. 154–76). New York, NY: Wiley.

Provides, in the authors' words, 'a goal-based motivational alternative to the symptom-centered, stage change models of human adjustment that have dominated clinical science.'

Martre, P. J., Dahl, K., Jensen, R., & Nordahl, H. M. (2013). Working with goals in therapy. In E. A. Locke & G. P. Latham (Eds.), *New developments in goal setting and task performance* (pp. 474–94). New York, NY: Routledge.

Provides updated literature on psychotherapy goal-setting.

Poulsen, A. A., Ziviani, J., & Cuskelly, M. (Eds.) (2015). *Goal setting and motivation in therapy: Engaging children and parents.* London, UK: Jessica Kingsley Publishers.

Excellent chapters addressing methods of collaborative goal-setting with child clients and their parents.

Winston, A., Rosenthal, R. N., & Pinsker, H. (2004). *Introduction to supportive psychotherapy. Core competencies in psychotherapy.* Arlington, VA: American Psychiatric Publishing.

Research-based guide for novice therapists that provides basic principles of psychotherapy that include realistic goal-setting with clients. Good case illustrations.

References

Abrines-Jaume, N., Midgley, N., Hopkins, K., Hoffman, J., Martin, K., Law, D., & Wolpert, M. (2016). A qualitative analysis of implementing shared decision making in child and adolescent mental health services in the United Kingdom: Stages and facilitators. *Clinical Child Psychology and Psychiatry, 21,* 19–31. doi: 10.1177/1359104514547596

Auerbach, S. M., May, J. C., Stevens, M., & Kiesler, D. J. (2008). Interactive role of working alliance and counselor-client interpersonal behaviors in adolescent substance abuse treatment. *International Journal of Clinical and Health Psychology, 8,* 617–29.

Bachelor, A. (2013). Clients' and therapists' views of the therapeutic alliance: Similarities, differences, and relationship to therapy outcome. *Clinical Psychology and Psychotherapy, 20,* 118–35. doi: 10.1002/cpp.792

Bachelor, A., Laverdière, O., Gamache, D., & Bordeleau, V. (2007). Clients' collaboration in therapy: Self-perceptions and relationships with client psychological functioning, interpersonal relations, and motivations. *Psychotherapy, Theory, Research, Practice, Training, 44,* 175–92. doi: 10.1037/0033-3204.44.2.175

Barkham, M., Mellor-Clark, J., Connell, J., & Cahill, J. (2006). A core approach to practice-based evidence: A brief history of the origins and applications of the CORE-OM and the CORE system. *Counselling and Psychotherapy Research, 6,* 3–15. doi: 10.1080/14733140600581218

Berking, M., Grosse Holtforth, M., Jacobi, C., & Kröner-Herwig, B. (2005). Empirically based goal-finding procedures in psychotherapy: Are some goals easier to attain than others? *Psychotherapy Research, 15,* 316–24. doi: 10.1080/10503300500091801

Brookman-Frazee, L., Haine, R. A., Gabayan, E. N., & Garland, A. F. (2008). Predicting frequency of treatment visits in community-based youth psychotherapy. *Psychological Services, 5,* 126–38. doi: 10.1037/1541-1559.5.2.126

Brunstein, J., Schultheiss, O., & Maier, G. W. (1999). The pursuit of personal goals: A motivational approach to well-being and life adjustment. In J. Brandstädter (Ed.), *Action self-development: Theory and research through the life span* (pp. 169–96). Thousand Oaks, CA: Sage.

Coatsworth, J. D., Santisteban, D. A., McBride, C. K., & Szapocznik, J. (2001). Brief strategic family therapy versus community control: Engagement, retention, and an exploration of the moderating role of adolescent symptom severity. *Family Process, 40,* 313–32. doi: 10.1111/j.1545-5300.2001.4030100313

Cohen, J. (1992). A power primer. *Psychological Bulletin, 112,* 155–9. doi: 10.1037/ 0033-2909.112.1.155

Cooper, M. & McLeod, J. (2007). A pluralistic framework for counselling and psychotherapy: Implications for research. *Counselling and Psychotherapy Research, 7,* 135–43. doi: 10.1080/14733140701566282

Cooper, M., Rowland, N., McArthur, K., Pattison, S., Cromarty, K., & Richards, K. (2010). Randomised controlled trial of school-based humanistic counselling for emotional distress in young people: Feasibility study and preliminary indications of efficacy. *Child and Adolescent Psychiatry and Mental Health, 4,* 1–12.

Creed, T. A., & Kendall, P. C. (2005). Therapist alliance building behavior within a cognitive-behavioral treatment for anxiety in youth. *Journal of Consulting and Clinical Psychology, 73,* 498–505. doi: 10.1037/0022-006X.73.3.498

Davidson, K., Perry, A., & Bell, L. (2015). Would continuous feedback of patient's clinical outcomes to practitioners improve NHS psychological therapy services? Critical analysis and assessment of quality of existing studies. *Psychology and Psychotherapy: Theory, Research and Practice, 88,* 21–37. doi: 10.1111/papt.12032

DeFife, J. A., & Hilsenroth, M. J. (2011). Starting off on the right foot: Common factor elements in early psychotherapy process. *Journal of Psychotherapy Integration, 21,* 172–91. doi: 10.1037/a0023889

Diamond, G. M., Liddle, H. A., Hogue, A., & Dakof, G. A. (1999). Alliance-building interventions with adolescents in family therapy: A process study. *Psychotherapy, 36,* 355–68. doi: 10.1037/h0087729

Dickson, J. M., & MacLeod, A. K. (2004). Approach and avoidance goals and plans: Their relationship to anxiety and depression. *Cognitive Therapy and Research, 28,* 415–32. doi: 10.1023/B:COTR.0000031809.20488.ee

Duncan, B. (2012). The Partners for Change Outcome Management System (PCOMS): The heart and soul of change project. *Canadian Psychology, 53,* 93–104. doi: 10.1037/ a0027762

Duncan, B. L., & Reese, R. J. (2015). The Partners for Change Outcome Management System: Revisiting the client's frame of reference. *Psychotherapy, 52,* 391––401. doi: 10.1037/pst0000026

Edbrooke-Childs, J., Jacob, J., Law, D., Deighton, J., & Wolpert, M. (2015). Interpreting standardized and idiographic outcomes measures in CAMHS: What does change mean and how does it relate to functioning and experience? *Child and Adolescent Mental Health, 20,* 142–8. doi: 10.1111/camh.12107

Elliot, A. J., & Church, M. A. (2002). Client-articulated avoidance goals in the therapy context. *Journal of Counseling Psychology, 49,* 243–54. doi: 10.1037/0022-0167.49.2.243

Emmons, R. A. (2003). Personal goals, life meaning, and virtue: Wellsprings of a positive life. In C. L. M. Keys & J. Haidt (Eds.), *Positive psychology and life well lived* (pp. 105–28). Washington, DC: American Psychological Association.

Faw, L., Hogue, A., Johnson, S., Diamond, G. M., & Liddle, H. A. (2005). The Adolescent Therapeutic Alliance Scale (ATAS): Initial psychometrics and prediction of outcome in family-based substance abuse prevention counseling. *Psychotherapy Research, 15,* 141–54. doi: 10.1080/10503300512331326994

Freund, A. M., & Riediger, M. (2006). Goals as building blocks of personality and development in adulthood. In D. K. Mroczek & T. D. Little (Eds.), *Handbook of personality development* (pp. 353–72). Mahwah, NJ: Erlbaum.

Garland, A. F., Hawley, K. M., Brookman-Frazee, L., & Hurlburt, M. S. (2008). Identifying common elements of evidence-based psychosocial treatments for children's disruptive behavior problems. *Journal of the American Academy of Child and Adolescent Psychotherapy, 47,* 505–14. doi: 10.1097/CHI.0b013e31816765c2

Garland, A. F, Lewczyk-Boxmeyer, C. M., Gabayan, E. N., & Hawley K. M. (2004). Multiple stakeholder agreement on desired outcomes for adolescents' mental health services. *Psychiatric Services, 55,* 671–6.

Goldman, R. E., Hilsenroth, M. E., Owen, J. J., & Gold, J. R. (2013). Psychotherapy and alliance: Use of cognitive-behavioral techniques within a short-term psychodynamic treatment model. *Journal of Psychotherapy Integration, 23,* 373–85. doi: 10.1037/a0034363

Gondek, D., Edbrooke-Childs, J., Fink, E., Deighton, J., & Wolpert, M. (2016). Feedback from outcome measures and treatment effectiveness, treatment efficiency, and collaborative practice: A systematic review. *Administration and Policy in Mental Health and Mental Health Services, 43,* 325–43. doi: 10.1007/s10488-015-0710-5

Grosse Holtforth, M., Bents, H., Mauler, B., & Grawe, K. (2006). Interpersonal distress as a mediator between avoidance goals and goal satisfaction in psychotherapy inpatients. *Clinical Psychology and Psychotherapy, 13,* 172–82. doi: 10.1002/cpp.486

Grosse Holtforth, M., & Castonguay, L. G. (2005). Relationship and techniques in cognitive-behavioral therapy—A motivational approach. *Psychotherapy: Theory, Research, Practice, Training, 42,* 443–55. doi: 10.1037/0033-3204.42.4.443

Grosse Holtforth M., & Grawe K. (2002). Bern Inventory of Treatment Goals: Part 1. Development and first application of a taxonomy of treatment goal themes. *Psychotherapy Research, 12,* 79–99. doi: 10.1080/71386961

Grosse Holtforth, M., Grawe, K., Egger, O., & Berking, M. (2005). Reducing the dread: Change of avoidance motivation in psychotherapy. *Psychotherapy Research, 15,* 261–71. doi: 10.1080/10503300512331334968

Grosse Holtforth, M., Reubi, I., Ruckstuhl, L., Berking, M. & Grawe, K. (2004). The value of treatment goal themes for treatment planning and outcome evaluation of psychiatric inpatients. *International Journal of Social Psychiatry, 50,* 80–91. doi: 10.1177/0020764004040955

Grossoehme, D. H., & Gerbetz, L. (2004). Adolescent perceptions of meaningfulness in psychiatric hospitalization. *Clinical Child Psychology and Psychiatry, 4,* 589–96. doi: 10.1177/1359104504046162

Harkin, B., Webb, T. L., Chang, B. P. I., Prestwich, A., Conner, M., Kellar, I., Benn, Y., & Sheeran, P. (2016). Does monitoring goal progress promote goal attainment? A meta-analysis of the experimental evidence. *Psychological Bulletin, 142,* 198–229. doi: 10.1037/bul0000025

Hawley, K. M., & Weisz, J. R. (2003). Child, parent, and therapist (dis)agreement on target problems in outpatient therapy: The therapist's dilemma and its implications. *Journal of Consulting and Clinical Psychology*, *71*, 62–70. doi: 10.1037/0022-006X.71.1.62

Hoong, S., Heathfield, H., Fitzpatrick, K., & Benson, L. (2014). *Closing the gap through changing relationships: Evaluation.* London: Office for Public Management. Retrieved from http://www.health.org.uk/publications/closing-the-gap-through-changing-relationships-evaluation/

Horvath, A. O., & Greenberg, L. S. (1989). Development and validation of the Working Alliance Inventory. *Journal of Counseling Psychology*, *36*, 223–33. doi: 10.1037/0022-0167.36.2.223

Jansson, B., Than, K., & Ramnerö, J. (2015). A structured approach to goal formulation in psychotherapy: Differences between patients and controls. *International Journal of Psychology and Psychotherapy*, *15*, 181–90.

Karver, M. S., Handelsman, J. B., Fields, S., & Bickman, L. (2006). Meta-analysis of therapeutic relationship variables in youth and family therapy: The evidence for different relationship variables in the child and adolescent treatment outcome literature. *Clinical Psychology Review*, *26*, 50–65. doi: 10.1016/j.cpr.2005.09.001

Lambert, M. (2010). *Prevention of treatment failure: The use of measuring, monitoring, and feedback in clinical practice.* Washington, DC: American Psychological Association. doi: 10.1037/12141-000

Lambert, M. J., & Shimokawa, K. (2011). Collecting client feedback. *Psychotherapy*, *48*, 72–9. doi: 10.1037/a0022238

Law, D., & Jacob, J. (2013). *Goals and goal based outcomes (GBOs): Some useful information.* Third Edition. CAMHS Press: London. Retrieved from https://www.researchgate.net/profile/Duncan_Law/publication/277868914

Law, D., & Wolpert, M. (2014). *Guide to using outcomes and feedback tools with children, young people, and families.* Retrieved from https://www.researchgate.net/publication/277870071

Lucock, M., Halstead, J., Leach, C., Barkham, M., Tucker, S., Randal, C., Middleton, J, Khan, W., Catlow, H., Waters, E., & Saxon, D. (2015). A mixed-method investigation of patient monitoring and enhanced feedback in routine practice: Barriers and facilitators. *Psychotherapy Research*, *25*, 633–46. doi: 101080/10503307.2015.1051163

Marmar, C. R., Horowitz, M. J., Weiss, D. S., & Marziali, E. (1989). The Development of the Therapeutic Alliance Rating System. In L. S. Greenberg & W. M. Pinsof (Eds.), *The psychotherapeutic process: A research handbook* (pp. 367–90). New York: Guilford Press.

McArthur, K., Cooper, M., & Berdondini, L. (2013). School-based humanistic counseling for psychological distress in young people: Pilot randomized controlled trial. *Psychotherapy Research*, *23*, 355–65. doi: 10.1080/10503307.2012.726750

McLeod, B. D. (2011). Relation of the alliance and outcomes in youth psychotherapy: A meta-analysis. *Clinical Psychology Review*, *37*, 603–16. doi: 10.1016/j.cpr.2011.02.001

Michalak, J., & Grosse Holtforth, M. (2006). Where do we go from here? The goal perspective in psychotherapy. *Clinical Psychology: Science and Practice*, *13*, 346–65. doi: 10.1111/j.1468-2850.2006.00048.x

Michalak, J., Klapphack, M. A., & Kosfelder, J. (2004). Personal goals of psychotherapy patients: The intensity and the "why" of goal-motivated behavior and their implications for therapeutic process. *Psychotherapy Research*, *14*, 193–209. doi: 10.1093/ptr/kph017

Norcross, J. C., & Wampold, B. E. (2011). Evidence-based relationships: Research conclusions and clinical practices. *Psychotherapy, 48*, 98–102. doi: 10.1037/a0022161

Parker-Pope, T. (2016, January 5). Develop a whole new you. *The New York Times*, p. D4.

Pereira, T., Lock, J., & Oggins, J. (2006). Role of the therapeutic alliance in family therapy for anorexia nervosa. *International Journal of Eating Disorders, 39*, 677–84. doi: 10.1002/eat

Proctor, G., & Hargate, R. (2013). Quantitative and qualitative analysis of a set of goal attainment forms in primary care mental health services. *Counseling and Psychotherapy Research, 13*, 235–41. doi: 10.1080/14733145.2012.742918

Pybis, J., Cooper, M., Hill, A., Cromarty, K., Levesley, R., Murdoch, J., & Turner, N. (2014). Pilot randomized controlled trial of school-based humanistic counselling for psychological distress in young people: Outcomes and methodological reflections. *Counselling and Psychotherapy Research.* doi: 10.1080/14733145.2014.905614

Roth, B. (2015). *The achievement habit: Stop wishing, start doing, and take command of your life.* New York, NY: Harper Business

Ryan, R. M., & Deci, E. L. (2008). A self-determination theory approach to psychotherapy: The motivational basis for effective change. *Canadian Psychology, 49*, 186–93. doi: 10.1037/a0012753

Ryan, R. M., Lynch, M. F., Vansteenkiste, M., & Deci, E. L. (2011). Motivation and autonomy in counseling, psychotherapy, and behavior change: A look at theory and practice. *The Counseling Psychologist, 39*, 193–260. doi: 10.1177/0011000009359313

Ryan, R. M., Plant, R. W., & O'Malley, S. (1995). Initial motivations for alcohol treatment: Relations with patient characteristics, treatment involvement, and dropout. *Addictive Behaviors, 20*, 279–97. doi: 10.1016/0306-4603(94)00072-7

Schulte-Bahrenberg, T., & Schulte, D. (1993). Change of psychotherapy goals as a process of resignation. *Psychotherapy Research, 3*, 153–65. doi: 10.1080/10503309312331333759

Shefler, G., Canetti, L., & Wiseman, H. (2001). Psychometric properties of goal-attainment scaling in the assessment of Mann's time-limited psychotherapy. *Journal of Clinical Psychology, 57*, 971–9. doi: 10.1002/jclp.1063

Shirk, S. R., Karver, M. S., & Brown, R. (2011). The alliance in child and adolescent psychotherapy. *Psychotherapy, 48*, 17–24. doi: 10.1037/a0022181

Stafford, V., Hutchby, I., Karim, K., & O'Reilly, M. (2016). "Why are you here?" Seeking children's accounts of their presentation to Child and Adolescent Mental Health Services (CAMHS). *Clinical Child Psychology and Psychiatry, 21*, 3–18. Doi: 10.1177/1359104514543957

Swift, J., & Callahan, J. (2009). Early psychotherapy processes: An examination of client and trainee clinician perspective convergence. *Clinical Psychology and Psychotherapy, 16*, 228–36. doi: 10.1002/cpp.617

Tracey, T. J., & Kokotovic, A. M. (1989). Factor structure of the Working Alliance Inventory. *Psychological Assessment, 1*, 207–10. doi: 10.1037/1040-3590.1.3.207

Tryon, G. S., & Winograd, G. (2011). Goal consensus and collaboration. *Psychotherapy, 48*, 50–7. doi: 10.1037/a0022061

Weisz, J. R., Chorpita, B. F., Frye, A., Ng, M. Y., Lau, N., Bearman, S. K., Ugueto, A.M., Langer, D.A., Hoagwood, K.E.; Research Network on Youth Mental Health (2011). Youth top problems: Using idiographic, consumer-guided assessment to identify treatment needs and to track change during psychotherapy. *Journal of Consulting and Clinical Psychology, 79,* 369–80. doi: 10.1037/a0023307

Wollburg, E., & Braukhaus, C. (2010). Goal-setting in psychotherapy: The relevance of approach and avoidance goals for treatment outcome. *Psychotherapy Research, 20,* 488–94. doi: 10.1080/10503301003796839

Wolpert, A., Ford, T., Trustam, E., Law, D., Deighton, J., Flannery, H., & Fugard, R. J. B. (2012). Patient-reported outcomes in child and adolescent mental health services (CAMHS): Use of idiographic and standardized measures. *Journal of Mental Health, 21,* 165–73. doi: 10.3109/09638237.2012.664304

Yeh, M., & Weisz, J. R. (2001). Why are we here at the clinic? Parent-child (dis)agreement on referral problems at outpatient treatment entry. *Journal of Consulting and Clinical Psychology, 69,* 1018–25. doi: 10.1037//0022-006X.69.6.1018

Zane, N., Sue, S., Chang, J., Huang, L., Huang, J., Lowe, S., Srinivasan, S., Chun, K., Kurasaki, K., Lee, E. (2005). Beyond ethnic match: Effects of client-therapist cognitive match in problem perception, coping orientation, and therapy goals on treatment outcomes. *Journal of Community Psychology, 33,* 569–85. doi: 10.1002/jcop.20067

Chapter 6

Measuring outcomes using goals

Jenna Jacob, Julian Edbrooke-Childs,
Christopher Lloyd, Daniel Hayes,
Isabelle Whelan, Miranda Wolpert,
and Duncan Law

The goals of this chapter are to:

◆ identify and review different goal-based outcome measures for children and adults;

◆ outline the considerations around psychometric properties of goal-based outcome measures;

◆ explain the benefits and challenges of goal-setting and tracking.

Goal-based measures

A direct focus on clients' goals was identified as a key aspect of effective care many years ago (Frank, 1973), and goal-setting has been used in therapy for several decades (e.g. Strupp & Hadley, 1977; Urwin, 2007). Setting goals in treatment helps to make the desired endpoint of therapy clearer, by setting out immediate tasks to contribute towards the ultimate aspiration (Austin & Vancouver, 1996; Goodman, 2001; Karoly, 1993; Locke & Latham, 1990). Tracking goals may also be useful as a self-regulation strategy, particularly when used to check against progress on a regular basis (Harkin et al., 2016). Goals can be areas agreed on to work towards and to be reviewed at the end of an intervention, without necessarily being explicitly routinely scored or tracked throughout (e.g. Randall & McEwen, 2000).

In response to the need to systematically track and monitor goals, goal attainment scaling (GAS; Kiresuk & Sherman, 1968) was developed in the late 1960s and continues to be used in a wide range of adult and child health settings. This measure sought to be more specific than the global 'goal met/not met' method of measurement, sometimes referred to as the 'checklist approach' that often accompanies goal-setting (Hurn, 2006).

Goals are a common framework against which people are able to measure their own success and progress. It is important to emphasize that goal-based outcome measures have not only been developed within the psychological literature but also within counselling and psychotherapy domains, as well as wider interdisciplinary fields, such as occupational health. Goals, aims, and targets have also historically been used in educational and organizational settings. For example, Achievement Goal Questionnaire (Finney, Pieper, & Barron, 2004), Target Complaints (Ames, 1992; Battle, Imber, Hoehn-Saric, Nash, & Frank, 1966), and SMART goals (Doran, 1981; Lawlor & Hornyak, 2012) have been used to measure outcomes for patients for some time in physical health (e.g. Farrand & Woodford, 2013; Schwartz & Drotar, 2006) and occupational health (e.g. Canadian Occupational Performance Measure; Law *et al.*, 1990). Goals have long been used in substance abuse treatment, with a focus on abstinence and relapse prevention from those seeking treatment (DuPont, 2014).

Research in relation to mental health has tended to focus on adult treatment goals (see Clare *et al.*, 2010; e.g. CORE Goal Attainment Form; CORE, 2016). Research on treatment goals in therapy with children and young people is a more recent development. However, the GAS (Kiresuk & Sherman, 1968), Goal Based Outcomes (GBO; Law, 2006), and Top Problems (Weisz *et al.*, 2011) have been used internationally with children in paediatric (Steenbeek, 2011) and mental health settings (Ruble, McGrew, & Toland, 2012) (see also CORC, 2015).

This process of tracking goals with measures is best exemplified by direct examples. The Goals Form, developed by Cooper (2015), is one such personalized tool that can be used to evaluate clients' goals within the therapeutic context, with both adults and children (see Figure 6.1). With this particular measure, clients are invited to set and agree between two and seven goals with their therapists in a first or second assessment session. For each individual goal, clients are then requested to specify how much they presently feel they have achieved it by circling a number from 1 (not at all achieved) to 7 (completely achieved).

Contextualizing different goal-based approaches

Within the Improving Access to Psychological Therapies (IAPT) agendas and across mental health services more broadly, substantive demand has been placed on practitioners and service providers to provide and report upon detailed and rigorous evidence of their clinical effectiveness. This has typically taken place within the form of standardized, problem-based measures (e.g. PHQ-9, GAD-7, BDI-II, SDQ, RCADS). In the section that follows we highlight some core distinctions that exist between different types of goal-based approaches, with both adults and children.

Client code:	Therapist:	Date:	Session:

Goals Form

Goal 1:

Not at all achieved						Completely achieved
1	2	3	4	5	6	7

Goal 2:

Not at all achieved						Completely achieved
1	2	3	4	5	6	7

Fig. 6.1 The Goals Form.

Source: Reproduced from Cooper, *The Goals Form: Guidance on use*, 2015, University of Roehampton, DOI: 10.13140/RG.2.1.2576.7767. This work is licensed under a Creative Commons Attribution-NoDerivatives 4.0 International licence. It is attributed to Mick Cooper and the original version can be found here: https://www.researchgate.net/publication/286928866_Goals_Form.

One longstanding distinction within the goal literature is between standardized (or 'nomothetic') and 'idiographic' measures of outcomes (Edbrooke-Childs, Jacob, Law, Deighton, & Wolpert, 2015). As mentioned above, while standardized measures have typically held prominence within research and clinical practice, idiographic goal measures, such as the Goal Based Outcome tool (Law, 2006) or Goal Attainment Scaling (Kiresuk & Sherman, 1968), can be developed by service users to suit their specific difficulties, or areas that they and the clinician feel should be the focus of an intervention. They are therefore sometimes seen as better at capturing change that is most relevant to service users themselves.

In contrast, standardized measures are general measures of mental health difficulties; for example, the Strengths and Difficulties Questionnaire (SDQ; Goodman, 1997) or the Patient Health Questionnaire (PHQ9). These generally have demonstrable psychometric evidence of their validity and reliability. However, within the complex milieu of mental health practice, these standardized measures of client outcomes have been criticized for failing to take account of the often idiographic and hence deeply subjective problems or areas for development which clients bring into the therapeutic context (Bromley & Westwood, 2013; Dozois, Dobson, & Ahnberg, 1998; Evans & Huxley, 2002; Hurn, 2006; Norman, Dean, Hansford, & Ford, 2013; Ruble *et al.*, 2012). In this sense, they have tended to represent broadly focused or predefined global statements, which are based on data aggregated from large samples. Furthermore, they tend to emphasize problems as opposed to goals; the former being difficulties or obstacles that clients wish to overcome, the latter about what the person is striving for. It has also been argued that standardized measures generally focus on symptomatology, and neglect other domains such as coping skills, which are particularly pertinent when working with individuals whose symptoms may not improve (Batty *et al.*, 2013). In this regard, standardized measures are often more broadly oriented, whereas idiographic measures are more focused (see Table 6.1). Nonetheless, standardized measures may have some greater utility over idiographic measures when aggregating data across groups of clients and examining change in outcomes at the level of a service, rather than for an individual.

A further distinction in the goals literature lies in approach versus avoidance goals (Eliot & Sheldon, 1997) (see Chapter 3, this volume). Typically, goals derived from many outcome measures, including standardized and idiographic instruments, can be classified as avoidance based. Such instances of avoidance-based goals might include wording goals around negative terms, such as: 'I want to stop eating too much sugar-based food' or 'I want to stop shouting at my kids'. As can be seen from these two examples, the specific wording in each of these goals suggests a desire to avoid, or move away from, a particular behaviour. Approach-based goals, however, tend to fit more congruently

Table 6.1 A four-way differential comparison of different goal dimensions

The nature of goals		
	Idiographic	**Nomothetic/standardized**
	◆ Focus on individual experience ◆ Does not compare individual against population norms ◆ Wording is created by client and therefore deeply personal and relevant ◆ Asserts importance of moving towards a goal	◆ Highly structured ◆ Evaluates individual against a standard population ◆ Assumed to measure standardized constructs, which are common to general population ◆ Wording is more generalized, global, and less specific to the individual, often focusing on reducing specific symptomatology
Approach	e.g. I want to learn to become more assertive with peers	e.g. I generally feel I want to be more positive about my life
Avoidance	e.g. I want to stop being unassertive with peers	e.g. I feel I want to be less depressed

with an idiographic methodology, often reflecting the socio-historical roots of anti-positivistic thinking, which has historically tended to place more emphasis on human flourishing as opposed to distress. Examples might include: 'I want to build a better relationship with my parents' or 'I want to build up my self-confidence at school'. Pertinent examples of approach-based goal measures for both adults and children can be found within the appendix to this chapter and further clarification of different goal-based dimensions is available in Table 6.1. Note, our review in the Appendix covers only those measures in which respondents were asked to identify goals, which were approach based in nature—rather than avoidant and/or problem focused. This decision was made largely owing to the paucity of research which presently covers their clinical utility within the literature. That is to say, measures in which the person is asked to specify what they would like to achieve, rather than overcome, have generally been overlooked within the literature.

Although the differences between approach and avoidance goals may seem only semantic, the literature has demonstrated deeper differences (see Chapter 3, this volume). Research has shown that clients who direct their attention to states that they wish to avoid in the therapeutic context (i.e. avoidance goal regulation) are more susceptible to negative processes and outcomes. Meanwhile, Elliot and Church (2002) showed that clients who adopted more avoidance goals in therapy showed smaller changes in wellbeing, experienced less progress towards goals, and were, overall, less satisfied with the work undertaken in therapy. These differences suggest a need to focus attention not only towards idiographic measures but also on helping clients to set goals which are approach based and personally meaningful.

Psychometric properties of goal-based measures

A variety of goal-setting outcome measures are commonly used in healthcare settings, such as Top Problems (used in child mental health in the USA; Weisz *et al.*, 2011), Target Complaints (Battle *et al.*, 1966), and the Clinical Outcomes in Routine Evaluation (CORE) Goal Attainment Form (used in adult mental health services in England; Proctor & Hargate, 2013). Goal attainment scaling (Kiresuk & Sherman, 1968) is widely used in child physical health settings (Steenbeek, 2011) and to a lesser extent in child mental health settings, in particular with children with conduct disorder (Maher & Barbrack, 1984) and autism spectrum disorder (Ruble *et al.*, 2012). As mentioned, the GBO tool (Law, 2006) is widely used for monitoring goals in child mental health services in England. With this measure, clinicians, young people, and carers, either independently or, ideally jointly, agree on their goals and rate progress towards achieving these over the course of treatment. We will be focusing on this measure in depth. Appendix 6.1 has further information on the psychometric properties of other goal-setting measures.

A study by Edbrooke-Childs *et al.* (2015) examined change in standardized and idiographic outcome measures in child mental health services, comparing change in progress towards goals with clinician-reported change (as measured by the Children's Global Assessment Scale, CGAS) and parent-reported satisfaction with care (as measured by the Experience of Service Questionnaire, ESQ). This was analysed against the associations between the change as measured by the standardized SDQ. Change in progress towards goals showed more significant associations with clinician-reported change and satisfaction with care, than did change in the SDQ. The relationships between goal progress and change in CGAS and satisfaction with care were also consistently stronger than the relationships between change in the SDQ and change in CGAS and satisfaction with care.

These findings also support the psychometric properties of the GBO. The GBO's internal consistency was acceptable, suggesting that ratings of progress towards goals may relate to the same underlying construct, even for different people's individually chosen goals (Edbrooke-Childs *et al.*, 2015). Furthermore, the GBO's reliable change index was 2.45 points (Edbrooke-Childs *et al.*, 2015), which suggests that change greater than this is unlikely to be solely attributable to measurement error (Jacobson & Truax, 1991). With regard to reviewing progress towards goals, if a young person has moved more than 2.45 points, researchers and clinicians can conclude that this is unlikely to result from fluctuations of measurement error alone.

Benefits of setting and tracking goals

There are myriad benefits to setting and tracking goals in therapy, from giving clients a sense of agency and personalization to the value for the practitioner in focusing, monitoring, and directing treatment and, indeed, in contributing to their own development as professionals.

Adults and children alike who receive support for mental health and wellbeing difficulties may value tracking their own goal progress, mainly because it supports collaboration with the healthcare professionals (Liberman & Kopelowicz, 2002; Moran, Kelesidi, Guglani, Davidson, & Ford, 2012). Individual mental health difficulties require individual outcome tracking; this has been reiterated by service users themselves (Badham, 2011).

At the simplest level, goal-tracking, alongside other measures of outcomes, helps to monitor progress. Clinicians have suggested that, without goal-setting, it can be easy to lose track of progress (Batty *et al.*, 2013; Pender, Tinwell, Marsh, & Cowell, 2013). As discussed, explicit goal-setting may offer an insight into areas of importance to the individual that may not be otherwise captured and measured in a systematic way. Further to this, evidence also suggests that goal-tracking can provide a focus for all involved to work together towards reaching common, concrete, and measureable objectives (Bromley & Westwood, 2013). Goal-tracking may also assist communication. It may be particularly useful in multidisciplinary working and for providing a different source of information about a case, from the user themselves (Emanuel, Catty, Anscombe, Cantle, & Muller, 2013).

Explicit goal-setting has also been shown to both motivate and engage service users to feel more involved in discussions about their care (Law & Wolpert, 2014). If monitoring shows that there is not progress towards a goal, discussions with the individual about their perception of the reasons for this and consolidating those with the practitioner's views may help to move therapy on or take a different direction. It has also been shown that parents of children who have set goals are more likely to be satisfied with the care received (Jacob *et al.*, 2017), which may be because of the personalized nature of goal-tracking.

Discussions about progress towards clients' goals, and use of other measures of outcome, can also aid supervision (Law & Jacob, 2015). Such measures can add valuable insight and concrete examples of areas to discuss in supervision meetings, and provide an opportunity to explore progress and other potential ways of working to assist the client to work towards meeting their goals.

Goal-setting and monitoring may be an important component of collaborative working with clients accessing services, and a key part of engaging their agency and involvement in their self-management. The personalized goals agreed in collaboration with professionals are a key component of precision mental health (Bickman, Kelley, Breda, de Andrade, & Riemer, 2011; Bickman, Lyon, & Wolpert, 2016; Carlier *et al.*, 2012; Knaup, Koesters, Schoefer, Becker, & Puschner, 2009; Lambert & Shimokawa, 2011). Working with user-defined goals may be particularly important in terms of therapy outcomes in child mental health and even more so with some of the most vulnerable groups, such as looked-after children, and those with experiences of abuse or neglect, where issues of epistemic trust may be crucial to engagement and outcomes (Bateman & Fonagy, 2016).

Setting and measuring to direct interventions and care decisions is central to a 'person-centred focus', which may lead to better shared decision making, communication, and therapeutic outcomes (Asarnow *et al.*, 2009; Kazdin, 1977;

Mulley, Trimble, & Elwyn, 2012; Westermann, Verheij, Winkens, Verhulst, & Van Ort, 2013), and has been advocated by service users and clinical academics (Chewning *et al.*, 2012; Reuben & Tinetti, 2012). Working out what goals to measure, and making them measurable, as well as personalized, is often one of the early pieces of collaborative work undertaken by clients, other close family members, and clinicians. This will usually begin with understanding what each of the parties believes to be the presenting problem (CORE, 2016; Law & Jacob, 2015). However, when more than two parties are involved, there may be different perceptions of what is wrong (Hawley & Weisz, 2003; Yeh & Weisz, 2001), and deliberation, negotiation, and facilitation are needed by the clinician to know what needs to be measured, and how to proceed. Alternatively, clients and other family members may come with many goals, in which case the role of the clinician is to help understand which ones are the most important to pursue in therapy (Law & Jacob, 2015). In such instances, the setting of up to three goals is suggested as good practice (Farrand & Woodford, 2013; Law & Jacob, 2015).

The move towards personalization reflects the need for client values to be taken into account in all aspects of care and treatment (Institute of Medicine, 2001). Setting and measuring goals can form a central component of this (Law & Jacob, 2015). However, while values and goals are closely linked, goals tend to include qualities such as being specific and measurable, whereas values are broader in concept and scope (Eccles & Wigfield, 2002). Although it may be easy to determine the client's and family's values and preferences, translating these into goals can sometimes prove challenging. Clients may struggle at first with aligning goals with SMART aims (Doran, 1981), a framework which allows clients to effectively define aims, as well as to measure and track progress over time (Doran, 1981). The clinician, through active client participation, can help with setting measurable goals, facilitating this through techniques such as motivational interviewing and solution-focused therapy with the client and family members. This process fits well with the aim of developing personalized goals, and draws on processes such as discussing self-efficacy, information exchange, and mutual agreement, which sit within shared decision making and person-centred care (Da Silva, 2012; Makoul & Clayman, 2006).

The use of personalized goals in therapy may also protect against a culture of 'tick box' exercises, which has become associated with standardized outcome measurement (Badham, 2011; Wolpert, Fugard, Deighton, & Görzig, 2012). Common barriers and objections from clinicians and service users relate to more standardized outcome measures not being applicable during therapy sessions, because of their content, the process of using the measure during sessions, or how the data from the measure are used (Wolpert, Curtis-Tyler, &

Edbrooke-Childs, 2016), with clinicians referring to standardized measures as impersonal (Norman *et al.*, 2013). Goal-based outcomes make this personal to the client through involving them in the deliberative process (Austin & Vancouver, 1996), measuring change over time based on what the client wants to achieve, including areas such as coping, confidence, and understanding—these are areas often missed through more standardized measurement (Jacob, Edbrooke-Childs, Law, & Wolpert, 2015), or when it may not be expected for a client to show improvement in symptoms. Recent research has tried to provide a framework for goal-based outcomes and standardized measurement, analysing the content of goals and identifying corresponding standardized measures (Jacob *et al.*, 2015). However, this work is still in its infancy, and not all goals have been matched onto standardized measures.

Challenges of setting and tracking goals

The challenges of measuring outcomes generally in mental health settings have been widely discussed (e.g. Fleming, Jones, Bradley, & Wolpert, 2016; Jacob *et al.*, in press; Wolpert *et al.*, 2016).

One potential limitation within mental health settings is the capacity of the client to be involved in treatment, let alone actively collaborate with a healthcare professional. This may be the case particularly when dealing with severe mental health difficulties (Hamann *et al.*, 2009; Seale, Chaplin, Lelliott, & Quirk, 2006) or when dealing with young people who may be deemed 'doubly incapacitated' by age and mental health difficulties (Fonagy, Steele, Steele, Moran, & Higgitt, 1991; Ruhe, Wangmo, Badarau, Elger, & Niggli, 2015). However, taking a skilled shared decision making approach, can enable some goal-setting even with clients deemed to have limited capacity.

Another challenge is the need to consider multiple stakeholders' views. This is a particularly acute issue with young people and parents, and also comes into play with other vulnerable groups, such as elderly clients or those with carers. The challenges may appear to be universal, but we draw on research in the child mental health field to demonstrate that disagreement between stakeholders is often high, which may contribute to poorer outcomes (Yeh & Weisz, 2001).

Some argue that measuring goals in mental health contexts is more challenging than in other areas because of the complex nature of mental health difficulties (as opposed to monitoring 'harder' outcomes such as deaths in surgery, for example, although these are also widely contested outcomes (Wolpert *et al.*, 2014)).

Others have argued that it is precisely the individual nature of these measures that leaves them more open to subjective interpretation, particularly if linked to performance targets (Bevan & Hood, 2006; Law, 2011). A further concern from service user advocates is that 'achieving' a goal could lead to termination of treatment (Moran *et al.*, 2012).

Other challenges include practical barriers such as inadequate IT systems and lack of resources; more individual factors such as personal views, beliefs, and preferences; and service factors such as regional and national target setting. Learning collaborations such as the Child Outcomes Research Consortium (CORC) and Children and Young People's Improving Access to Psychological Therapies (CYP IAPT); (Law & Wolpert, 2014) support clinicians and services to work through these barriers to ensure the appropriate use of measures and data.

Concerns over the lack of adequate IT systems to record and track goals throughout therapy (Fleming *et al.*, 2016) can be countered by arguing that all that is needed to track a goal on a scale between 0 and 7 or 0 and 10 is a pen and paper. One of the reasons that it may not be possible to record the scores from goals into an existing IT system may be because the relevant service or trust is committed to using other, more standardized, measures of outcome to demonstrate movement towards set targets.

Specific arguments that highlight the challenges of goal-setting and tracking (including tracking all outcomes) with children and young people include concerns over very young children's capacity to understand their own mental health because of their age, but this is also confounded by mental health difficulties (e.g. autism, Baron-Cohen, Leslie, & Frith, 1985). However, the use of goal-setting in child mental health settings has been found to be likely with younger, rather than older, children and it has been suggested that it is helpful for young children who are below the lower age limit for some more standardized measures of outcome (Jacob *et al.*, 2017), perhaps because of these comprehension difficulties.

Practitioners can also have a mistrust of personalized outcomes in terms of striking a balance between the involvement of the child/young person and their vulnerability (Abrines-Jaume *et al.*, 2016; Wolpert *et al.*, 2014). However, appropriate training and highlighting the benefits of using goals may dispel some of these concerns. Service users themselves can be well placed to increase buy-in from practitioners, by emphasizing the value they have found from using goals (for examples, see Law & Wolpert, 2014).

Conclusion

We have outlined here research on the use and tracking of goals. Good evidence has been found for the use of goal-setting and monitoring with both adults and children. The flexible and global nature of goals mean that there does not appear to be a need for separate measures for adults and children, and lessons can be learnt from all settings and population groups. The most straightforward way to track outcomes using goals is as discussed: to ask people what are their goals of therapy, and how close they are to meeting those goals and using that as a starting point. The scoring system used to then track the progress of the goals that have been set becomes secondary, particularly to clinical practice. There may be more imaginative work to be done when setting goals with children as opposed to adults, and perhaps more guidance from parents and clinicians. Clinicians may also want to consider the impact of multiple stakeholders on the scoring and tracking of goals.

Goal-tracking has been used for some time but it is now being explored in more detail in child mental health settings, particularly as a key component of personalized care. The suggestion is to use goals as a basis to think about what areas of outcome are the most important for that individual to measure and that it may also be helpful to track goals, particularly where symptoms are not expected to improve. The psychometric evidence available has been discussed and offers support for the validity of goals as a method of tracking outcomes information. Good face validity among service users and clinicians also strengthens the argument for systematic monitoring and measuring of goals.

Because recovery means different things to different people, goal-setting provides an opportunity for children and young people to express what this might look like to them and to share this insight with their families and the professionals working with them. It may be that there is some work to be done to agree on goals in child mental health settings and it may also require some abstract thinking about the remit of the work being done, and how that can still go some way towards meeting the goals that have been set.

We have also discussed some of the challenges to measuring goals and how these are perhaps outweighed by the benefits shown by previous research, including giving clients ownership of their care, providing a focus for clinicians and service users, and being a source of useful information for clinicians' supervision. It is our view that goal measurement and tracking should be central to the therapy process, to ensure that the outcomes being tracked are important to the individual, whether they are an adult or a child; the adaptability of goals allows for this crossover.

Points for reflection

♦ If you think that outcome measures should be used, do you think idiographic measures such as goal-setting and tracking should be used instead of, or in addition to, standardized measures?

- ◆ Can you think of any cases in which goal-setting and tracking would be beneficial? Can you think of any cases in which goal-setting and tracking would be less useful? What are the key differences between these types of cases?
- ◆ How do you think goals that young people set might differ from those set by carers or therapists, and how would you try to align any differences?

Further reading

Carlier, I. V. E., Meuldijk, D., Van Vliet, I. M., Van Fenema, E., Van der Wee, N. J. A., & Zitman, G. (2012). Routine outcome monitoring and feedback on physical or mental health status: evidence and theory. *Journal of Evaluation in Clinical Practice*, *18*(1), 104–10. doi: 10.1111/j.13652753.2010.01543.x

Farrand, P., & Woodford, J. (2013). *Goal Setting in Low Intensity CBT*. Exeter, UK: CEDAR, University of Exeter.

Hurn, J., Kneebone, I., & Cropley, M. (2006). Goal setting as an outcome measure: a systematic review. *Clinical Rehabilitation*, *20*, 756–72.

Jacob, J., Edbrooke-Childs, J., Holley, S., Law, D., & Wolpert, M. (2015). Horses for courses? A qualitative exploration of goals formulated in mental health settings by young people, parents, and clinicians. *Clinical Child Psychology and Psychiatry*, *21*(2), 208–23. doi: 10.1177/1359104515577487.

Law, D. & Jacob, J. (2015). *Goals and Goal Based Outcomes (GBOs): some useful information* (3rd ed.). London: CAMHS Press.

Proctor, G., & Hargate, R. (2013). Quantitative and qualitative analysis of a set of goal attainment forms in primary care mental health services. *Counselling and Psychotherapy Research*, *13*(3), 235–241. doi: 10.1080/14733145.2012.742918

References

Abrines-Jaume, N., Midgley, N., Hopkins, K., Hoffman, J., Martin, K., Law, D., & Wolpert, M. (2016). A qualitative analysis of implementing shared decision making in Child and Adolescent Mental Health Services in the United Kingdom: Stages and facilitators. *Clinical Child Psychology and Psychiatry*, *21*(1), 19–31. doi: 10.1177/1359104514547596

Ames, C. (1992). Classrooms: goals, structures and student motivation. *Journal of Educational Psychology*, *84*(3), 261–71.

Asarnow, J. R., Jaycox, L. H., Tang, L., Duan, N., LaBorde, A., Zeledon, L., Anderson, M., Murray, P. J., Landon, C., Rea, M. M., Wells, K. B. (2009). Long-term benefits of short-term quality improvement interventions for depressed youths in primary care. *American Journal of Psychiatry*, *166*(9), 1002–10. doi: 10.1176/appi.ajp.2009.08121909

Austin, J. T., & Vancouver, J. B. (1996). Goal constructs in psychology: Structure, process, and content. *Psychological Bulletin*, *120*(3), 338–75. doi: 10.1037/0033-2909.120.3.338

Badham, B. (2011). *Talking about talking therapies: thinking and planning about how to make good and accessible talking therapies available to children and young people.* London: YoungMinds.

Baron-Cohen, S., Leslie, A. M., & Frith, U. (1985). Does the autistic child have a "theory of mind"? *Cognition*, *21*(1), 37–46. doi: 10.1016/0010-0277(85)90022-8

Bateman, A. W., & Fonagy, P. (2016). *Mentalization-Based Treatment for Personality Disorders: A Practical Guide.* Oxford: Oxford University Press.

Battle, C. C., Imber, S. D., Hoehn-Saric, R., Nash, E. R., & Frank, J. D. (1966). Target complaints as criteria of improvement. *American Journal of Psychotherapy, 20*(1), 184–92.

Batty, M. J., Moldavsky, M., Foroushani, P. S., Pass, S., Marriott, M., Sayal, K., & Hollis, C. (2013). Implementing routine outcome measures in child and adolescent mental health services: from present to future practice. *Child and Adolescent Mental Health, 18*(2), 82–7. doi: 10.1111/j.1475-3588.2012.00658.x

Bevan, G., & Hood, C. (2006). What's measured is what matters: targets and gaming in the English public health care system. *Public Administration, 84*(3), 517–38. doi: 10.1111/j.1467-9299.2006.00600.x

Bickman, L., Kelley, S. D., Breda, C., de Andrade, A. R., & Riemer, M. (2011). Effects of routine feedback to clinicians on mental health outcomes of youths: results of a randomized trial. *Psychiatric Services, 62*(12), 1423–9. doi: 10.1176/appi.ps.002052011

Bickman, L., Lyon, A. R., & Wolpert, M. (2016). Achieving precision mental health through effective assessment, monitoring, and feedback processes: introduction to the special issue. *Administration and Policy in Mental Health and Mental Health Services Research,* 271-6. doi: 10.1007/s10488-016-0718-5

Bromley, C., & Westwood, S. (2013). Young people's participation: views from young people on using goals. *Clinical and Family Psychology Review, 1,* 41–60.

Carlier, I. V. E., Meuldijk, D., Van Vliet, I. M., Van Fenema, E., Van der Wee, N. J. A., & Zitman, F. G. (2012). Routine outcome monitoring and feedback on physical or mental health status: evidence and theory. *Journal of Evaluation in Clinical Practice, 18*(1), 104–10. doi: 10.1111/j.1365-2753.2010.01543.x

Chewning, B., Bylund, C. L., Shah, B., Arora, N. K., Gueguen, J. A., & Makoul, G. (2012). Patient preferences for shared decisions: a systematic review. *Patient Education and Counseling, 86*(1), 9–18. doi: 10.1016/j.pec.2011.02.004

Clare, L., Linden, D. E. J., Woods, R. T., Whitaker, R., Evans, S. J., Parkinson, C. H., van Paasschen J, Nelis SM, Hoare Z, Yuen KS, Rugg, M. D. (2010). Goal-oriented cognitive rehabilitation for people with early-stage Alzheimer disease: a single-blind randomized controlled trial of clinical efficacy. *The American Journal of Geriatric Psychiatry, 18*(10), 928–39. doi: 10.1097/JGP.0b013e3181d5792a

Cooper, M. (2015). The Goals Form. University of Roehampton. London. Retrieved from https://www.researchgate.net/publication/286928866_Goals_Form (Accessed 26 April 2017)

CORC. (2015). Homepage, from http://www.corc.uk.net/

CORE. (2016). Goal Attainment Form, from http://www.coreims.co.uk/About_Measurement_CORE_Tools.html

Da Silva, D. (2012). *Evidence: Helping people share decision making. A review of evidence considering whether shared decision making is worthwhile.* London: The Health Foundation.

Doran, G. T. (1981). There's a SMART way to write management's goals and objectives. *Management Review, 70*(11), 35–6.

Dozois, D. J., Dobson, K. S., & Ahnberg, J. L. (1998). A psychometric evaluation of the Beck Depression Inventory–II. *Psychological assessment, 10*(2), 83.

DuPont, R. L. (2014). *Creating a New Standard for Addiction Treatment Outcomes*. Report from the Institute for Behavior and Health, Inc.

Eccles, J. S., & Wigfield, A. (2002). Motivational beliefs, values, and goals. *Annual Review of Psychology, 53*(1), 109–32.

Edbrooke-Childs, J., Jacob, J., Law, D., Deighton, J., & Wolpert, M. (2015). Interpreting standardized and idiographic outcome measures in CAMHS: what does change mean and how does it relate to functioning and experience? *Child and Adolescent Mental Health, 20*(3), 142–8. doi: 10.1111/camh.12107

Elliot, A. J., & Church, M. A. (2002). Client articulated avoidance goals in the therapy context. *Journal of Counseling Psychology, 49*(2), 243–54.

Eliot, A. J., & Sheldon, B. (1997). Avoidance achievement motivation: a personal goals analysis. *Journal of Personality and Social Psychology, 73*(1), 171.

Emanuel, R., Catty, J., Anscombe, E., Cantle, A., & Muller, H. (2014). Implementing an aim-based outcome measure in a psychoanalytic child psychotherapy service: Insights, experiences and evidence. *Clinical Child Psychology and Psychiatry, 19*(2), 169-83. doi: 10.1177/1359104513485081

Evans, S., & Huxley, P. (2002). Studies of quality of life in the general population. *International Review of Psychiatry, 14*(3), 203–11.

Farrand, P., & Woodford, J. (2013). *Goal Setting in Low Intensity CBT*. Exeter, UK: CEDAR, University of Exeter.

Finney, S. J., Pieper, S. L., & Barron, K. E. (2004). Examining the Psychometric Properties of the Achievement Goal Questionnaire in a General Academic Context. *Educational and Psychological Measurement, 64*(2), 365–82. doi: 10.1177/0013164403258465

Fleming, I., Jones, M., Bradley, J., & Wolpert, M. (2016). Learning from a learning collaboration: the CORC approach to combining research, evaluation and practice in child mental health. *Administration and Policy in Mental Health and Mental Health Services Research, 43*(3), 297–301. doi: 10.1007/s10488-014-0592-y

Fonagy, P., Steele, M., Steele, H., Moran, G. S., & Higgitt, A. C. (1991). The capacity for understanding mental states: the reflective self in parent and child and its significance for security of attachment. *Infant Mental Health Journal 12*(3), 201–18.

Frank, J. D. (1973). *Persuasion and healing: A comparative study of psychotherapy*. New York, NY: Schoken.

Goodman, R. (1997). The Strengths and Difficulties Questionnaire: a research note. *Journal of Child Psychology and Psychiatry, 38*(5), 581–6. doi: 10.1111/j.1469-7610.1997.tb01545.x

Goodman, R. (2001). Psychometric properties of the Strengths and Difficulties Questionnaire. *Journal of the American Academy of Child and Adolescent Psychiatry, 40*(11), 1337–45. doi: 10.1097/00004583-200111000-00015

Hamann, J., Mendel, R., Cohen, R., Heres, S., Ziegler, M., Bühner, M., & Kissling, W. (2009). Psychiatrists' use of shared decision making in the treatment of schizophrenia: patient characteristics and decision topics. *Psychiatric Services (Washington, D.C.), 60*(8), 1107–12.

Harkin, B., Webb, T., L., Chang, B., P. I., Prestwich, A., Conner, M., Kellar, I., Benn, Y., Sheeran, P. (2016). Does monitoring goal progress promote goal attainment? A meta-analysis of the experimental evidence. *Psychological Bulletin, 142*(2), 198–229.

Hawley, K. M., & Weisz, J. R. (2003). Child, parent, and therapist (dis)agreement on target problems in outpatient therapy: the therapist's dilemma and its implications. *Journal of Consulting and Clinical Psychology, 71*(1), 62–70. doi: 10.1037/0022-006X.71.1.62

Hurn, J., Kneebone, I., & Cropley, M. (2006). Goal setting as an outcome measure: a systematic review. *Clinical Rehabilitation, 20,* 756–72.

Institute of Medicine. (2001). *Crossing the quality chasm: A new health system for the 21st century.* Washington DC: National Academy Press.

Jacob, J., De Francesco, D., Deighton, J., Law, D., Wolpert, M., & Edbrooke-Childs, J. (2017). Goal formulation in child mental health settings: when is it more likely and is it associated with satisfaction with care? *European Child and Adolescent Psychiatry, 26*(7), 759-70. doi: 10.1007/s00787-016-0938-y

Jacob, J., Edbrooke-Childs, J., Law, D., & Wolpert, M. (2015). Measuring what matters to patients: using goal content to inform measure choice and development. *Clinical Child Psychology and Psychiatry, 22*(2), 170-86. doi: 10.1177/1359104515615642

Jacob, J., Napoleone, E., Zamperoni, V., Levy, L., Barnard, M., & Wolpert, M. (2017). How can outcome data inform change? Experiences from the child mental health context in Great Britain, including barriers and facilitators to the collection and use of data. In T. Tilden & B. E. Wampold (Eds.), *Routine Outcome Monitoring in Couple and Family Therapy* (pp. 261–279). Cham, Switzerland: Springer International Limited.

Jacobson, N. S., & Truax, P. (1991). Clinical significance: A statistical approach to defining meaningful change in psychotherapy research. *Journal of Consulting and Clinical Psychology, 59*(1), 12–19.

Karoly, P. (1993). Goal systems: an organizing framework for clinical assessment and treatment planning. *Psychological Assessment, 5*(3), 273–80.

Kazdin, A. E. (1977). Assessing the Clinical or Applied Importance of Behavior Change through Social Validation. *Behavior Modification, 1*(4), 427–52. doi: 10.1177/014544557714001

Kiresuk, T. J., & Sherman, R. E. (1968). Goal attainment scaling: A general method for evaluating comprehensive community mental health programs. *Community Mental Health Journal, 4*(6), 443–53. doi: 10.1007/BF01530764

Knaup, C., Koesters, M., Schoefer, D., Becker, T., & Puschner, B. (2009). Effect of feedback of treatment outcome in specialist mental healthcare: Meta-analysis. *The British Journal of Psychiatry, 195*(1), 15–22.

Lambert, M. J., & Shimokawa, K. (2011). Collecting client feedback. *Psychotherapy, 48*(1), 72–9.

Law, D. (2006). *Goal Based Outcomes (GBOs): some useful information.* Retrieved from www.corc.uk.net

Law, D. (2011). *Goals and Goal Based Outcomes (GBOs): some useful information.* London: CAMHS Press.

Law, D., & Jacob, J. (2015). *Goals and Goal Based Outcomes (GBOs): some useful information (3rd ed.).* London: CAMHS Press.

Law, D., & Wolpert, M. (Eds.). (2014). *Guide to Using Outcomes and Feedback Tools With Children, Young People and Families* (2nd ed.). London: CAMHS Press.

Law, M., Baptiste, S., McColl, M., Opzoomer, A., Polatajko, H., & Pollock, N. (1990). The Canadian occupational performance measure: an outcome measure for occupational therapy. *Canadian Journal of Occupational Therapy, 57*(2), 82–7. doi: 10.1177/000841749005700207

Lawlor, K. B., & Hornyak, M. J. (2012). Smart goals: How the application of smart goals can contribute to achievement of student learning outcomes. *Developments in Business Simulation and Experiential Learning, 39*, 259–67.

Liberman, R. P., & Kopelowicz, A. (2002). Rehab rounds: teaching persons with severe mental disabilities to be their own case managers. *Psychiatric Services, 53*(11), 1377–9. doi: 10.1176/appi.ps.53.11.1377

Locke, E. A., & Latham, G. P. (1990). *A theory of goal setting and task performance.* Englewood Cliff, NH: Prentice-Hall.

Maher, C. A., & Barbrack, C. R. (1984). Evaluating the individual counseling of conduct problem adolescents: the goal attainment scaling method. *Journal of School Psychology, 22*, 285–97.

Makoul, G., & Clayman, M. L. (2006). An integrative model of shared decision making in medical encounters. *Patient Education and Counseling, 60*(3), 301–12. doi: 10.1016/j.pec.2005.06.010

Moran, P., Kelesidi, K., Guglani, S., Davidson, S., & Ford, T. (2012). What do parents and carers think about routine outcome measures and their use? A focus group study of CAMHS attenders. *Clinical Child Psychology and Psychiatry, 17*(1), 65–79. doi: 10.1177/1359104510391859

Mulley, A. G., Trimble, C., & Elwyn, G. (2012). Stop the silent misdiagnosis: Patients' preferences matter. *BMJ, 345*, e6572. doi: 10.1136/bmj.e6572

Norman, S., Dean, S., Hansford, L., & Ford, T. (2013). Clinical practitioners' attitudes towards the use of Routine Outcome Monitoring within Child and Adolescent Mental Health Services: A qualitative study of two Child and Adolescent Mental Health Services. *Clinical Child Psychology and Psychiatry, 19*(4), 576–95. doi: 10.1177/1359104513492348

Pender, F., Tinwell, C., Marsh, E., & Cowell, V. (2013). Evaluating the use of goal-based outcomes as a single patient rated outcome measure across CWP CAMHS: a pilot study. *Child and Family Clinical Psychology Review, 1*, 29–40.

Proctor, G., & Hargate, R. (2013). Quantitative and qualitative analysis of a set of goal attainment forms in primary care mental health services. *Counselling and Psychotherapy Research, 13*(3), 235–41. doi: 10.1080/14733145.2012.742918

Randall, K. E., & McEwen, I. R. (2000). Writing patient-centered functional goals. *Physical Therapy, 80*(12), 1197–203.

Reuben, D. B., & Tinetti, M. E. (2012). Goal-oriented patient care—an alternative health outcomes paradigm. *New England Journal of Medicine, 366*(9), 777–9. doi: 10.1056/NEJMp1113631

Ruble, L., McGrew, J. H., & Toland, M. D. (2012). Goal attainment scaling as an outcome measure in randomized controlled trials of psychosocial interventions in autism. *Journal of Autism and Developmental Disorders, 42*(9), 1974–83. doi: 10.1007/s10803-012-1446-7

Ruhe, K. M., Wangmo, T., Badarau, D. O., Elger, B. S., & Niggli, F. (2015). Decision-making capacity of children and adolescents—suggestions for advancing the concept's implementation in pediatric healthcare. *European Journal of Pediatrics*, *174*(6), 775–82. doi: 10.1007/s00431-014-2462-8

Schwartz, L., & Drotar, D. (2006). Defining the nature and impact of goals in children and adolescents with a chronic health condition: a review of research and a theoretical framework. *Journal of Clinical Psychology in Medical Settings*, *13*(4), 390–402. doi: 10.1007/s10880-006-9041-8

Seale, C., Chaplin, R., Lelliott, P., & Quirk, A. (2006). Sharing decisions in consultations involving anti-psychotic medication: a qualitative study of psychiatrists' experiences. *Social Science & Medicine*, *62*(11), 2861–73.

Steenbeek, D., Gorter, J.W., Ketelaar, M., Galama, K. & Lineman, E. (2011). Responsiveness of Goal Attainment Scaling in comparison to two standardized measures in outcome evaluation of children with cerebral palsy. *Clinical Rehabilitation*, *25*(12), 1128–39.

Strupp, H. H., & Hadley, S. W. (1977). A tripartite model of mental health and therapeutic outcomes: With special reference to negative effects in psychotherapy. *American Psychologist*, *32*(3), 187–96.

Urwin, C. (2007). Revisiting 'What works for whom?': A qualitative framework for evaluating clinical effectiveness in child psychotherapy. *Journal of Child Psychotherapy*, *33*(2), 134–60. doi: 10.1080/00754170701431370

Weisz, J. R., Chorpita, B. F., Frye, A., Ng, M. Y., Lau, N., Bearman, S. K., Ugueto, A. M., Langer, D. A., Hoagwood, K. E.; Research Network on Youth Mental Health. (2011). Youth Top Problems: using idiographic, consumer-guided assessment to identify treatment needs and to track change during psychotherapy. *Journal of Consulting and Clinical Psychology*, *79*(3), 369–80. doi: 10.1037/a0023307

Westermann, G. M. A., Verheij, F., Winkens, B., Verhulst, F. C., & Van Ort, F. V. A. (2013). Structured shared decision-making using dialogue and visualization: a randomized controlled trial. *Patient Education and Counseling*, *90*(1), 74–81. doi: 10.1016/j.pec.2012.09.014

Wolpert, M., Curtis-Tyler, K., & Edbrooke-Childs, J. (2016). A qualitative exploration of patient and clinician views on Patient Reported Outcome Measures in child mental health and diabetes services. *Administration and Policy in Mental Health and Mental Health Services Research*, *43*(3), 309–15. doi: 10.1007/s10488-014-0586-9

Wolpert, M., Deighton, J., De Francesco, D., Martin, P., Fonagy, P., & Ford, T. (2014). From 'reckless' to 'mindful' in the use of outcome data to inform service-level performance management: perspectives from child mental health. *BMJ Quality & Safety*, *23*(4), 272–6. doi: 10.1136/bmjqs-2013-002557

Wolpert, M., Fugard, A. J. B., Deighton, J., & Görzig, A. (2012). Routine outcomes monitoring as part of children and young people's Improving Access to Psychological Therapies (CYP IAPT)—improving care or unhelpful burden? *Child and Adolescent Mental Health*, *17*(3), 129–30. doi: 10.1111/j.1475-3588.2012.00676.x

Yeh, M., & Weisz, J. R. (2001). Why are we here at the clinic? Parent-child (dis) agreement on referral problems at out-patient treatment entry. *Journal of Consulting and Clinical Psychology*, *69*, 1018–25. doi: 10.1037/0022-006X.69.6.1018

Appendix 6.1. Goal-based outcome measures for children and adults

Goal attainment scaling

Age range

Both young people and adults, who are capable of complex cognitive reasoning.

Description

Goal attainment scaling or GAS, as it is commonly abbreviated, was first developed by Kiresuk & Sherman (1968), as a collaborative interview-focused tool between client and therapist and remains one of the most widely adopted approaches to the measurement of personalized treatment goals in the therapeutic setting. GAS is intentionally broad in its remit and its strength lies in its general applicability to a broad range of clinical settings, with varying outcomes of interest. The use of GAS in the therapeutic alliance involves the client articulating general goals, which are subsequently scaled on a core evaluation system, which remain personally meaningful to the client yet are discernible to others beyond the therapeutic dyad.

Administration and scoring

Salient goals identified are placed onto a scale that ranges from least to most positive outcome. A minimum of 2 points on the scale should hold concrete and objective descriptions for the status of the client's progress to be readily understandable to other professionals. Subsequently, points on the scale are allocated numerical values (e.g. − 2 for the least favourable outcome, 0 for the most likely treatment outcome, and + 2 for the most favourable treatment outcome), to define a measurable yet meaningful scale for each goal. Generally, three to four goals are identified, which are then combined into the single GAS score. For further information on scoring with GAS, please consult the key reference.

Psychometric properties

Most of the psychometric data relating to GAS is concerned with wider health-care settings, with little attention thus far focused on mental health contexts. In settings in which psychometric properties have been established, GAS has demonstrated commendable scores: inter-rater reliability 0.87 (geriatric care; Stolee, Rockwood, Fox, & Streiner, 1992), 0.92 (brain injury rehabilitation; Joyce, Rockwood, & Mate-Kole, 1994), or 0.86 (Mann's time limited psychotherapy; Shefler, Canetti, & Wiseman, 2001). Inter-rater reliability refers to the degree to which GAS scores are consistent with each other over time. Validity for GAS, which suggests the extent to which GAS measures what it claims to measure, was also strong ($r = .81$ in brain injury rehabilitation; Joyce, Rockwood & Mate-Kole, 1994).

Key reference

Kiresuk, T. J., & Sherman, M. R. E. (1968). Goal attainment scaling: A general method for evaluating comprehensive community mental health programs. *Community Mental Health Journal*, 4(6), 443–53.

The CORE Goal Attainment Form (GAF)

Age range

Both young people and adults.

Description

The GAF is a derivative form of the CORE (Clinical Outcomes for Routine Evaluation) system (Evans *et al.*, 2000; see the CORE System User Manual: http://www.coreims.co.uk/). The GAF is a patient-centred satisfaction and evaluation tool, which allows change to be measured from the client's standpoint. GAF is purpose-designed to complement other nomothetic measures used under the CORE umbrella, such as the CORE-OM, by providing additional qualitative and idiosyncratic data pertaining to client goals and how they found the process of therapy. The use of GAF permits clients to articulate their own goals for therapy. The CORE Partnership particularly recommends the use of GAF in clients who do not demonstrate a clinical or reliable change on the CORE-OM. As noted earlier in Chapter 6, individualized measures are particularly sensitive when monitoring small yet meaningful levels of client change.

Administration and scoring

At the beginning of therapy clients are requested to pinpoint up to four foremost difficulties that they wish therapy to assist with. At the termination of therapy, the client is requested to complete side two of the form, which probes the degree to which they found therapy beneficial with each difficulty expressed (from 'Not at all' to 'Extremely'), and to provide further qualitative and quantitative feedback about the experience of therapy. Scoring is based on the magnitude of difference between pre-and post-treatment scores.

Psychometric properties

No studies currently exist which demonstrate the psychometric properties of GAF.

Key reference

Proctor, G., & Hargate, R. (2013). Quantitative and qualitative analysis of a set of goal attainment forms in primary care mental health services. *Counselling and Psychotherapy Research, 13*(3), 235–41.

The Goals Form

Age range

Both young people and adults.

Description

The Goals Form, developed by Cooper (2015), is a concise personalized tool that can be used to evaluate clients' progress towards goals in therapy. These goals should usually be agreed in a first or second assessment session and determined by clients, in partnership and discussion with therapists. The use of the Goals Form positions goal behaviours as fluid and, when using this measure, it should be explained to clients that goals can be revised, deleted, or supplemented during the course of therapy. The Goals Form is structured so that clients will usually establish between two and seven goals, in the first instance. The Goals Form places a strong emphasis on goals, which have clarity, and are based around 'approach' as opposed to 'avoidance' aims. More specifically, it is more useful if the client identifies an aim to achieve and move towards rather than to move away from. For each individual goal, clients should be requested to specify how much they presently feel they have achieved it by circling a number from 1 (Not at all achieved) to 7 (Completely achieved).

Administration and scoring

To calculate changes over the course of therapy and for service evaluation purposes, the authors of the Goals Form have created a systematic method for scoring. Please consult the key reference below.

Psychometric properties

Test-retest reliability from assessment to first session was .74, meaning the Goals Form was largely able to capture the same results across time.

In terms of convergent validity, the Goals Form showed a large significant correlation with the CORE-OM at baseline ($r = -.66$). More specifically, the concepts measured within the Goals Form strongly related to those measured within the CORE-OM.

Key reference

Cooper, M. (2015). *The Goals Form.* University of Roehampton. London. Retrieved from
   https://www.researchgate.net/publication/286928866_Goals_Form

Personal project analysis (PPA)

Age range

Both young people and adults.

Description

Personal project analysis, initially developed by Little (1983), is a highly adaptable multicomponent measure which can be used to decipher 'personal projects' of meaning for clients and to determine their subjective worth. It is derived from the psychology field but has the potential to be adapted for use in clinical practice. Personal projects are defined as activities undertaken over a period of time and in a specific social context, to attain an end named and given meaning by the client (Little, Salmela-Aro, & Philips, 2007). These can reflect past, current, and future single events, such as planning a holiday or ongoing tasks, such as completing a degree or maintaining fitness levels.

Administration and scoring

There are four stages of the PPA: elicitation, appraisal, hierarchy, and cross impact. In the elicitation stage, the model of personal projects is concisely introduced and the client is requested to compile a list of all their current projects. In the second appraisal stage, the client is asked to rate a core number of projects on features pertinent to the research or clinical situation. In the hierarchy module, the client identifies their underlying motivation for each project. In the cross impact stage, the client is requested to examine the effect of each project on the other projects (Little, 2011b). That is to say, the potential inter-relationship between each project is determined and reflected upon by the client.

Psychometric properties

The test–retest reliability of PPA, which refers to the level of consistency in results taken from the same individuals over a minimum of two periods of time, is moderate. Furthermore, high inter-rater agreement was found when coding project categories according to specific domains of activity. In terms of validity, independent associations between each of the PPA factors and measures of quality of life and clinical concerns such as depression have been found, lending support to the validity of the measure (Little, 2011a).

Key reference

Little, B. R., Salmela-Aro, K., & Phillips, S. D. (Eds.). (2007). *Personal project pursuit: Goals, action and human flourishing.* Mahwah, NJ: Lawrence Erlbaum Associates.

Selves Questionnaire (SQ)

Age range

Both young people and adults.

Description

The Selves Questionnaire (SQ; Higgins, Bond, Klein, & Strauman, 1986) is an open-ended interview measure, asking the client to articulate their principles (hopes and aspirations), which represent important promotion goals (Higgins, Shah, & Friedman, 1997). Participants are also asked to describe their actual self, their ideal self, and their 'ought' self in addition to their own beliefs and wider sensitivities of what significant others (e.g. a sibling, partner, or parent) would think about them. Later revised versions (Kinderman & Bentall, 1996) have extended the original format to include physical characteristics or representations of self but all still measure and view the magnitude of difference among the actual self, ideal self, and ought-self as paramount in locating psychological distress and areas of treatment in goal monitoring. It is derived from the psychology field but has the potential to be adapted for use in clinical practice.

Administration and scoring

Scoring is based on the client determining characteristics of self they currently possess (scaled from 1: not at all, to 10: strongly held) and would like to have (which can broadly be referred to as goals), which are then measured for a magnitude of difference.

Psychometric properties

The Selves Questionnaire (in both its original or modified form) has established its validity in a wide range of studies. Clinically depressed and socially phobic patients (Strauman, 1989) as well as clinically anxious and depressed students (Scott & O'Hara, 1993) have been shown to demonstrate specific patterns of discrepancies as predicted by the theoretical constructs underlying the Selves Questionnaire (Strauman & Higgins, 1988). The reliability of the modified Selves Questionnaire has been established in previous studies (Kinderman & Bentall, 1996). Inter-rater reliability, which refers to the degree of agreement between two independent clinicians, was high (= 0.985).

Key reference

Higgins, E. T., Bond, R. N., Klein, R., & Strauman, T. (1986). Self-discrepancies and emotional vulnerability: how magnitude, accessibility, and type of discrepancy influence affect. *Journal of Personality and Social Psychology*, 51(1), 5.

Intergoal Relations Questionnaire (IRQ)

Age range

Both young people and adults.

Description

The IRQ, developed by Riediger & Freund (2004), is an idiographic assessment tool which encourages the client to set personally meaningful goals and to reflect on the subsequent relationship between these goals. For instance, two separate goals might be associated insofar as advancement towards one goal might facilitate, prevent, or have an ambivalent effect on the other goal. The pursuit of the goal 'to gain muscle mass' might foster a positive influence on the goal 'to increase my physical strength'. It is possible, however, that two goals might contact conflicting essences in which the achievement of one goal deters the advancement of another. Hence, the IRQ supports clients to establish clear goals and, importantly, to consider their inter-relationship. It is derived from the psychology field but has the potential to be adapted for use in clinical practice.

Administration and scoring

Clients are asked to list qualitatively their current goals in succinct terms. Clients are then instructed to select three of these goals which are the most important to them, bracketing these off, respectively, as Goals A, B, and C. Clients then select a short keyword to refer to each goal; for example, 'fitness', 'confidence', 'family'. Each pair of two goals is then subjected to a series of six standardized questions, which encourages reflection on the inter-relationship between the goals in scaled terms. For example, 'because of the pursuit of Goal A', how likely is it on scale of 1–5 (with 1 being never and 5 being very often), that 'you do not invest as much time into Goal B as you would like to?'. This format continues for each paired goal and covers six domains: time, finance, energy, incompatible strategies, strategy overlap, and instrumental relations.

Psychometric properties

No available psychometric data.

Key reference

Riediger, M., & Freund, A. M. (2004). Interference and facilitation among personal goals: Differential associations with subjective well-being and persistent goal pursuit. *Personality and Social Psychology Bulletin, 30*(12), 1511–23.

Counselling Goals Systems (CoGS)

Age range

Children and young people (CYP) aged 11–25 years.

Description

CoGS was developed as an online interactive tool for CYP who used their counselling and support services online and face-to-face across 19 areas of the UK. It positions young people as autonomous agents in control of their goals and progress, affording them the ability to input defined, measurable, achievable, realistic, and timed personalized goals and to track them on a weekly basis.

Administration and scoring

During counselling, the practitioner supports the client to set and express their goals. The tasks that need to be carried out to attain these goals are then considered collaboratively, with the client scaling their progress towards achieving their own goal on scale of 1–10.

Psychometric properties

Not known.

Key reference

Sefi, A., & Hanley T. (2012). Examining the complexities of measuring effectiveness of online counselling for young people using routine evaluation data. *Pastoral Care in Education 30*(1): 49–64.

Goal Based Outcome (GBO) tool

Age range

Designed for use with children and young people (CYP) and families, with the lower age limit dependent on developmental ability, applicable across all ages. Useful with parents to rate their experience of child's progress towards goals.

Description

The GBO tool has been primarily developed to be used with children and young people, and their parents, but is applicable for use across all age ranges and abilities. It allows children and young people, and adults, as well as parents, to set agreed personalized goals for therapy and other psychological interventions and for service evaluation research. The tool has options for multiple perspective goal-setting, such as parents, other family members or carers, teachers, and other professionals.

Administration and scoring

Clients should be supported to set up to three goals collaboratively over the course of the first three sessions of the assessment or intervention. The client may select more goals but for outcome-related research, the top three should be selected by the client and subsequently ranked from 1 to 3. A score of 1 equates to the most prioritized by the client, with 3 being the least. For administrative purposes, it may be helpful if each goal is attached to an ID number. The client should then rate goals for current progress (T1). For example, from 0 to 10 where '0' means the goal is not met in any way and '10' means the goal is met completely. The scale has a midway anchor point rating of '5', which would indicate that the client feels they are halfway to reaching the goal. Coming to the end of the therapy or after six months, clients should repeat progress ratings (T2). It is optional whether goals are collected and collated in this time frame and there is the option to collect goal data from clients, during every session. Overall goal progress is calculated by subtracting the T1 score from the T2 score.

Psychometric properties

While data pertaining to the reliability of the GBO are not currently available, client progress towards goals appears to correlate with symptom improvement, as rated by both carers and clinical staff (Wolpert, Ford, *et al.*, 2012). This goes some way to demonstrating the overall validity of GBO. Good face validity, reliable change index = 3.

Key reference

Law, D. & Jacob, J. (2015). *Goals and Goal Based Outcomes (GBOs): some useful information (3rd ed.)*. London: CAMHS Press.

References

Cooper, M. (2015). *The Goals Form*. University of Roehampton, London. Retrieved from https://www.researchgate.net/publication/286928866_Goals_Form

Evans, C., Mellor-Clark, J., Margison, F., Barkham, M., Audin, K., Connell, J., & McGrath, G. (2000). CORE: clinical outcomes in routine evaluation. *Journal of Mental Health, 9*(3), 247–55.

Higgins, E. T., Bond, R. N., Klein, R., & Strauman, T. (1986). Self-discrepancies and emotional vulnerability: how magnitude, accessibility, and type of discrepancy influence affect. *Journal of Personality and Social Psychology, 51*(1), 5.

Higgins, E. T., Shah, J., & Friedman, R. (1997). Emotional responses to goal attainment: strength of regulatory focus as moderator. *Journal of Personality and Social Psychology, 72*(3), 515.

Joyce, B. M., Rockwood, K. J., & Mate-Kole, C. C. (1994). Use of goal attainment scaling in brain injury in a rehabilitation hospital. *American Journal of Physical Medicine & Rehabilitation, 73*(1), 10–14.

Kinderman, P., & Bentall, R. P. (1996). Self-discrepancies and persecutory delusions: evidence for a model of paranoid ideation. *Journal of Abnormal Psychology, 105*(1), 106.

Kiresuk, T. J., & Sherman, M. R. E. (1968). Goal attainment scaling: A general method for evaluating comprehensive community mental health programs. *Community Mental Health Journal, 4*(6), 443–53.

Law, D. & Jacob, J. (2015). *Goals and Goal Based Outcomes (GBOs): some useful information (3rd ed.)*. London: CAMHS Press.

Little, B. R. (1983). Personal projects: A rationale and method for investigation. *Environment and Behavior, 15*(3), 273–309.

Little, B. R. (2011a). Personal projects and motivational counselling: The quality of living reconsidered. In W. M. Cox & E. Klinger (Eds.), *Handbook of motivational counselling* (2nd ed., pp. 50–73). Chichester, UK: Wiley.

Little, B. R. (2011b). Personality science and the northern tilt: As positive as possible under the circumstances. In K. M. Sheldon, B. Kasdann, & M. F. Steger (Eds.), *Designing positive psychology: Taking stock and moving forward* (pp. 228–47). New York: Oxford University Press.

Little, B. R., Salmela-Aro, K. E., & Phillips, S. D. (2007). *Personal project pursuit: Goals, action, and human flourishing*. Mahwah, NJ: Lawrence Erlbaum Associates Publishers.

Proctor, G., & Hargate, R. (2013). Quantitative and qualitative analysis of a set of goal attainment forms in primary care mental health services. *Counselling and Psychotherapy Research, 13*(3), 235–41.

Riediger, M., & Freund, A. M. (2004). Interference and facilitation among personal goals: Differential associations with subjective well-being and persistent goal pursuit. *Personality and Social Psychology Bulletin, 30*(12), 1511–23.

Scott, L., & O'Hara, M. W. (1993). Self-discrepancies in clinically anxious and depressed university students. *Journal of Abnormal Psychology, 102*(2), 282.

Sefi, A., & Hanley, T. (2012). Examining the complexities of measuring effectiveness of online counselling for young people using routine evaluation data. *Pastoral Care in Education, 30*(1): 49–64.

Shefler, G., Canetti, L., & Wiseman, H. (2001). Psychometric properties of goal-attainment scaling in the assessment of Mann's time-limited psychotherapy. *Journal of Clinical Psychology, 57*(7), 971–9.

Stolee, P., Rockwood, K., Fox, R. A., & Streiner, D. L. (1992). The use of goal attainment scaling in a geriatric care setting. *Journal of the American Geriatrics Society, 40*(6), 574–8.

Strauman, T. J. (1989). Self-discrepancies in clinical depression and social phobia: Cognitive structures that underlie emotional disorders? *Journal of Abnormal Psychology, 98*(1), 14.

Strauman, T. J., & Higgins, E. T. (1988). Self-discrepancies as predictors of vulnerability to distinct syndromes of chronic emotional distress. *Journal of Personality, 56*(4), 685–707.

Wolpert, M., Ford, T., Trustam, E., Law, D., Deighton, J., Flannery, H., & Fugard, R. J. (2012). Patient-reported outcomes in child and adolescent mental health services (CAMHS): Use of idiographic and standardized measures. *Journal of Mental Health, 21*(2), 165–73.

Chapter 7

From problems to goals: Identifying 'good' goals in psychotherapy and counselling

Windy Dryden

Overview

The goals of this chapter are:

+ to outline what makes a 'good' goal in psychotherapy and counselling;

+ to argue that negotiating goals make most sense when a clear understanding has been arrived at concerning the psychological state of the client. Distinctions will be made among the psychological states of disturbance, dissatisfaction, and development. Goals can be negotiated with respect to each psychological state;

+ to identify and discuss various problems with respect to goals.

Alvin Mahrer (1967) edited one of the most seminal publications on goals in the field of psychotherapy where each contributor, a well-known figure in the field at that time, addressed the question, 'What are the goals of psychotherapy?'. In his concluding chapter, Mahrer reviewed what his contributors had to say on this issue and argued that two broad goals of psychotherapy could be identified from what they had written. These goals were the alleviation of suffering and the promotion of growth or development. It is important to note that the first of these goals refers to the absence of a psychological state (i.e. suffering), whereas the second refers to the presence of a state (i.e. growth or development). Thus, right from the outset, there was confusion concerning what constitutes a good goal in psychotherapy and counselling. Is it the absence of a negative psychological state, the presence of a positive psychological, state or both? Interestingly, this confusion also appears when clients are asked to nominate their therapeutic goals. In the present chapter, I will consider this issue and several others as I set out to achieve my primary chapter goal: to outline what makes a 'good' goal so that therapists can work effectively with goals in psychotherapy and counselling. Let me be clear at the outset that much of what I have to say is influenced by the theory underpinning rational emotive behaviour therapy (REBT). In my view, this theory has much to offer the subject of goals in psychotherapy and counselling and helps clarify a number of the issues that I will discuss in this chapter. When reading this chapter, please bear in mind that good goals are collaboratively negotiated between you and your client rather than unilaterally set and the more they are owned by the client, the more they are likely to be pursued and achieved (Law & Jacob, 2015).

Problems and goals

Let me begin with a very common scenario. A person seeks therapy from you because they have one or more psychological problems and want help with this problem or problems. The first step is for you to understand and help the client to understand the problem(s) for which they are seeking help.

Focus on the target problem

Let's suppose that you and your client decide to target one of your client's problems for therapeutic help. When this happens this problem is known as the 'target problem'.

When the target problem is assessed, if possible, you need to understand both a specific example of the target problem and its general nature.

AC-based problem focus.

Once a target problem has been selected and put in its general and specific context, then you need to engage with the client in the process of understanding the nature of the problem. In doing this here, I will use the 'A' and 'C' components of REBT's 'ABC' framework. 'A' stands for activating event and is divided into the Actual situation and what the person is most disturbed about—here known as the Adversity. 'C' (Consequences) stands for the emotional, behavioural, and cognitive responses to the adversity at 'A'. 'B' stands for Beliefs.

An example appears in the following box.

> Martha is anxious about an upcoming job interview. What she has most anxiety about is revealing her ignorance to the panel. The behavioural features of her anxiety are overpreparation for the interview, staying up all night rehearsing her answers, and avoiding eye contact in the interview. The cognitive features of her anxiety are thinking that the panel members will ask her any questions that she won't be able to answer and that the

members will think she is a complete idiot if she reveals her ignorance. Using the "ABC" framework:

A (Actual situation) = Job interview

(Adversity) = Revealing my ignorance

B (Beliefs) = Not known

C (Consequences)

(emotional) = Anxiety

(behavioural) = Overpreparation before the interview

= Avoiding eye contact during the interview

(cognitive) = "The panel members will ask me any questions I won't be able to answer"

= "The panel members will think I am a complete idiot if I show my ignorance"

Focus on goals

After you have helped yourself and your client to understand the 'A' (Actual situation and Adversity) and 'C' (Consequences) components of their target problem, you are in a good position to set a goal with respect to that problem.

Here are some examples of questions that you might ask to initiate this process:

◆ 'What would you take away from therapy that would give you a sense that you could effectively deal with the issue?'

◆ 'Instead of responding to the situation or adversity with [name the client's current problematic response], how would you like to be able to deal with it?'

◆ 'Instead of responding to the situation or adversity with [name the client's current problematic response], what would an acceptable constructive response be for you?'

The importance of negotiating a goal in response to the adversity rather than in response to the actual situation

Often when people discuss their problems in therapy they talk about their disturbed responses to the actual situations that they find problematic. Thus, as discussed in the Case example below, when one client first told me what he wanted to focus on in therapy, he said that he was anxious about giving presentations. When we looked further we found out what it was about giving presentations that made him most anxious: he thought that his Board of Directors would think that he was not up to the job. In the ABC framework, giving presentations was my client's Actual situation and thinking that his Board of Directors would think he was not up to the job was his Adversity.

If clients tend to identify actual situations when they nominate their target problem, they do the same when discussing their goal unless guided to set a goal with respect to their adversity. You will probably have to give them a rationale for providing such guidance, which they need to accept before you both proceed. Thus, you might ask them: 'Do you think it will be more useful if I help you to deal more productively with giving presentations or with the possibility that your Board of Directors may not think that you are up to the job, given the fact that the latter is what you are most anxious about?', or 'Do you think I can help you best with giving presentations if you are anxious about your Board of Directors thinking that you may not be up to the job or concerned, but not anxious about this?'.

The importance of assuming temporarily that your client's adversity is accurate

When your client comes to therapy struggling in the face of an adversity, therapy provides them with an opportunity to deal constructively with that adversity. In some forms of therapy, the emphasis is on helping clients to see that their inferred adversities at 'A's are distorted (e.g. 'my boss wants to see me because he wants to tell me off'), and that the thrust will be on helping them by questioning these distorted inferences. Although this stance is often useful, it does not help your client to deal constructively with adversity from their frame of reference. In addition, it is not inconceivable that they may encounter situations in which their inferences turn out to be correct. Thus, while my client may at times distort reality by assuming that people think negatively of him if he reveals gaps in his knowledge during a presentation, this may happen and, as such, it is important that you help him deal with this eventuality, assuming that he sees the sense of doing so. In encouraging your client to deal with the adversity from his frame of reference and thus to set goals for dealing with it constructively, it is useful to encourage your client to assume temporarily that he is accurate in inferring the presence of the adversity. The best time for a client to stand back and consider the accuracy or otherwise of his adversity inference is when he is not in a disturbed frame of mind about this inference, that is when he has achieved his goal of dealing constructively with the adversity. Thus, the client who thinks that her boss wants to see her to criticize her is better placed to consider the accuracy of this inference when she is concerned, but not anxious, about this inference, than when she is anxious about it.

Helping your client to construct healthy responses to the adversity as goals

Once your client understands the importance of negotiating a goal with respect to facing their adversity, then your next task is to help them to construct healthy responses to that adversity. These will serve as their goals with respect to their target problem. In my view, the best way to do this is to take the AC components that you identified when working to understand the problem. The 'A' components were the situation in which the problem occurred (the Actual situation) and what the client was most disturbed about (the Adversity). When negotiating a goal with the client, it is important to keep these 'A' components the same. Otherwise the client will not be helped to deal with their adversity constructively. The 'C' components are the emotional, behavioural, and cognitive responses to the adversity. In helping a client to construct healthy responses, ideally you need to help them identify alternative healthy responses to each of the unhealthy responses in the three response categories listed above, that is emotional, behavioural, and cognitive.

Healthy emotional responses as goals

When a person has a problem with an adversity, they usually experience a negative emotion. I call this negative emotion unhealthy when it leads the person to get stuck, is associated with a variety of unconstructive behavioural and cognitive responses, and discourages the person from facing up to and dealing constructively with the adversity. When the person responds constructively to the adversity they also experience a negative emotion. Why? Because the 'A' is negative and it is healthy to feel negative when something negative happens. I call this negative emotion healthy when it leads the person to get unstuck, is associated with a variety of constructive behavioural and cognitive responses and encourages the person to face up to and deal constructively with the adversity.

Negotiating a healthy emotional response to an adversity can often be quite difficult with a client as people generally think that such a response involves the diminution or absence of an unhealthy negative emotion rather than the presence of a healthy negative one. Also, in the English language we do not have terms that clearly denote healthy negative emotions in a way that clearly differentiate them from unhealthy negative emotions. Consequently, it is important that you negotiate with your client terms for both the unhealthy negative emotion that they experience in their target problem and their healthy negative emotion which they will experience if they reach their goal.

Healthy behavioural responses

Perhaps the easiest healthy responses to construct are behavioural in nature. As I will discuss below, it is important, if possible, to help the person nominate the presence of a healthy behaviour rather than the absence of an unhealthy behaviour.

Healthy cognitive responses

When constructing healthy cognitive responses to the adversity, that is responses that accompany emotions at 'C' rather than those that mediate (at 'B') responses to the adversity at 'A', a useful rule of thumb is as follows. Healthy cognitive responses are balanced and incorporate negative, neutral, and positive features of 'A' (e.g. 'Possibly being the laughing stock of the company and getting sacked, but more likely being helped to improve my performance and to rectify gaps in my knowledge'), whereas unhealthy cognitive responses are highly distorted and skewed to the negative (e.g. 'Being the laughing stock of the company and getting sacked').

Problems and goals: case example

Here is a case that I saw where my client's general target problem was 'I get anxious whenever I have to give a talk in public', and the specific example was 'I have to give a talk to the Board of Directors on Monday and I am anxious'. Below, is how I helped my client to understand the specific example of his target problem and then to set goals with respect to this target problem. I will provide explanatory commentary at various salient points.

Understanding the problem

CLIENT: I am anxious about giving a talk to the Board of Directors on Monday.

WD (AS THERAPIST): What's threatening to you about giving the talk?

[Here I use my knowledge that when a person is anxious it is because they are inferring the presence of something threatening to their personal domain at 'A'.]

CLIENT: I may reveal gaps in my knowledge and they may think that I am not up to the job.

WD: Are you most anxious about revealing gaps in your knowledge or the Directors thinking you are not up to the job?

CLIENT: The latter.

[I now have the actual situation and the adversity and can go on to explore the other 'C' aspects of the problem that accompany anxiety]

WD: What will you do or feel like doing before the talk and also during the talk when you are anxious?

[Having gotten the emotional component C (i.e. anxiety), I assess for the presence of the behavioural components of 'C'.]

CLIENT: Beforehand, I will do a lot of preparation and rehearsal and during the talk, I will avoid looking at the Directors and just concentrate on my PowerPoint slides

WD: And when you are anxious what do you tend to think?

[Now I am assessing for the presence of the cognitive components of 'C'.]

CLIENT: I think that I will be the laughing stock of the company and that they will sack me.

Here is a summary of the client's problem.

A (Actual Situation): Giving a talk to my Board of Directors

(Adversity): The Directors thinking that I am not up to the job

B (Beliefs): Not known yet

C (Consequences)

(emotional): Anxiety

(behavioural): Before giving the talk: overpreparation and over-rehearsal

During the talk: avoiding looking at the audience

(cognitive): Being the laughing stock of the company, getting sacked

---

Note that the 'B' section (which stands for beliefs) is not yet known. This section is assessed once the target problem and the goal with respect to that target problem have been identified and agreed. As such, it lies outside the scope of this chapter.

Negotiating goals

WD: So you are anxious about giving the talk on Monday and what you are most anxious about is that the Directors will think that you are not up to the job if you reveal gaps in your knowledge. Is that right?

CLIENT: Pretty much.

WD: What would you like to achieve in discussing this problem with me?

CLIENT: I would like to be able to be confident about giving the presentation.

[Here the client has nominated a positive psychological state with respect to his goal. However, note that he has not specified a goal concerning how to deal with the situation where the Directors might think that he is not up to the job. At the moment he would feel anxious about this possibility and he thinks that confidence is a good goal alternative to feeling anxious. So I have to do something tricky here: to work with the client's stated goal—to feel confident about giving the presentation—and to help him set a goal concerning the prospect that the Directors may think that he is not up to the job.]

Thus, it is important to help clients set goals in the face of adversity before helping them to reach their stated goals when these goals make no reference to the adversity in question. In the above example, I proceed thus:

wd: OK, so you would like to feel confident about giving presentations and I will certainly help you to do that. However, given that you feel anxious about the prospect of the Directors thinking that you are not up to the job, do you think that it would be wise if I first helped you to deal better emotionally about them thinking that?

CLIENT: But if I feel confident, then I will do a good job and then they won't think that I am not up to the job.

[Here, the client points out that if the adversity does not occur, he will have nothing to be anxious about. However, the grim reality is that I do not have the time to help the client develop the confidence that he is seeking. Such confidence will develop once the client has given several talks while dealing with the adversity of negative judgement in more productive ways. Thus, it is possible that the client will reveal gaps in his knowledge and it is possible that the Directors, or at least some of them, will think that he is not up to the job. So I need to help the client deal with the adversity given that I cannot help him avoid the adversity.]

wd: That's true and if I could help you develop the confidence that you want before Monday, I would, but how likely is it that you are going to go from being anxious to feeling confidence in one jump?

CLIENT: Not very likely.

wd: And even if you had the confidence that you seek, does that mean that you would not reveal gaps in your knowledge or that the Directors would not think that you were not up to the job?

CLIENT: No, I guess not.

wd: So given that, would you like me to help you deal more productively with the possibility that you may reveal gaps in your knowledge and that the Directors, or at least some of them, may think you are not up to the job?

CLIENT: Yes, that makes sense.

wd: So, I need to help you to experience an emotion which is negative given that for you the Directors thinking that you are not up to the job is negative, but one that helps you do the best job possible. Does that make sense?

CLIENT: Yes, it does.

WD: What emotion about the Directors thinking you are not up to the job would be negative in tone, would help you do the best job you could do?

CLIENT: To be less anxious than I am currently?

[Here the client comes up with a common response—he is in fact wanting to experience the same disturbed emotion, but with less intensity. REBT theory discriminates between an unhealthy negative emotion, like anxiety, and a healthy negative emotion, like concern. While unhealthy negative emotions have behavioural and cognitive referents that are unconstructive and tend to interfere with the person dealing effectively with the adversity in question (see the client's 'C' responses above), their healthy negative emotion counterparts have behavioural and cognitive referents that are constructive and tend to help the person deal effectively with the same adversity. My job is to help the client understand this difference and implement it in constructing a goal, in this case, concern rather than anxiety.]

WD: Actually, I may be able to do better than that. What if I could help you experience an emotion that was negative in tone, given that the Directors thinking you are not up to the job is negative, but one that has none of the unproductive behaviours and thinking associated with anxiety, one that helps you prepare sensibly, but not overprepare, one that leads to productive rehearsal, but not unproductive over-rehearsal and one that leads you to be more balanced in your thinking about the consequences of the Directors possibly thinking you are not up to the job, would you be interested in such an emotion?

CLIENT: Yes, definitely. What is it?

WD: It is un-anxious concern. Shall I help you to develop this emotion and its associated behaviours and thinking?

CLIENT: Yes, please.

The interested reader is directed to Dryden (2012) for more information concerning developing emotional goals together with their associated behavioural and thinking components.

AC-based goal focus

I mentioned above that the A (actual situation and adversity) and C (emotional, behavioural and cognitive consequences) components of the ABC framework drive the therapist's focus on the client's target problem. They also drive the therapist's focus on the client's goal with respect to that target problem. In doing so, the therapist ensures that the client sets a goal with respect to the adversity at 'A' rather than bypassing the 'A'. The therapist, in the above example, shows how to respond when the client tries to factor out the adversity in their goal-setting.

If the above therapist had used the AC components of the ABC framework in a formal way by putting their formulation with the above client's goal in written form it would be as follows:

A (Actual Situation): Giving a talk to my Board of Directors

(Adversity): The Directors thinking that I am not up to the job

B (Beliefs): Not known yet

C (Consequences)

(emotional goal): Concern

(behavioural goal): Before giving the talk: Sensible preparation rather than overpreparation; adequate rehearsal rather than over-rehearsal

During the talk: Looking at the audience

(cognitive goal): Possibly being the laughing stock of the company and getting sacked, but more likely being helped to improve my performance and rectify gaps in my knowledge

---

Note again that the 'B' section is not yet known. As, before this section is assessed once the target problem and the goal with respect to that target problem have been identified and agreed. Also note that the 'A' features are the same in both the problem and the goal (i.e. actual situation: Giving a talk to my Board of Directors, and adversity: The Directors thinking that I am not up to the job). This shows the importance that a good 'goal' is one that helps your client deal effectively with the problematic situation and what the person finds particularly aversive about the situation that makes it a problem for them. Given this, in addition to negotiating goals which are developmental or growthful in nature and which tend to bypass the adversity, it is important to help clients set goals that deal with this adversity. Generally speaking, if you attempt to help clients pursue their development or growth goals before helping them deal with adversity goals, the presence of the adversity will interfere with the work that you both plan to do in helping achieve the development goals.

Negotiating goals appropriate to your client's psychological state

So far in this chapter, I have stressed the importance of helping clients to set goals with respect to the adversities that they are actually facing, think they are facing, or predict that they will face.

Negotiating 'addressing disturbance' goals

My message has been that when clients are psychologically disturbed about these adversities, it is important to help them address this disturbance and to set goals which acknowledge that it is healthy to feel badly (but not disturbed) about the adversity and, indeed, doing so helps them face and deal with the adversity. REBT theory calls the emotional components of such disturbance 'unhealthy negative emotions' with the emotional components of their healthy emotional counterparts being referred to as 'healthy negative emotions'. Another way of looking at this is that while unhealthy negative emotions represent 'disturbance', healthy negative emotions represent 'dissatisfaction', realistic negative psychological states that are free from disturbance. I have already made the point that we do not have an agreed language for healthy negative emotions, but with this in mind Table 7.1 outlines common adversities, the unhealthy negative emotions or disturbance for which people seek help and the healthy negative emotions or dissatisfaction that form realistic emotional goals in the face of adversity.

Table 7.1 Common adversities, unhealthy negative emotions, or disturbance (Problems), and healthy negative emotions or dissatisfaction (Goals)

Adversity	Unhealthy negative emotions (disturbance): problem	Healthy negative emotions (dissatisfaction): goal
◆ Threat	Anxiety	Concern
◆ Loss ◆ Failure ◆ Undeserved plight (self or other)	Depression	Sadness
◆ Moral code violation ◆ Hurting others	Guilt	Remorse
◆ Falling very short of ideal ◆ Others negatively evaluate self	Shame	Disappointment
◆ Self more invested in relationship than is the other	Hurt	Sorrow
◆ Rule violation ◆ Threat to self-esteem ◆ Frustration	Unhealthy anger	Healthy anger
◆ Other poses threat to one's relationship	Unhealthy jealousy	Healthy jealousy
◆ Other has something that self prizes but does not have	Unhealthy envy	Healthy envy

I often sum up this position with clients by saying that I can help them feel badly about the adversities that they face and when they object by saying that are already feeling badly, I point out that they are actually feeling disturbed about the adversity and that I can help them take away the disturbance, but I can't help them take away their bad feelings, which are, as I point out a realistic and healthy responses to adversity!

I often find it valuable to 'unpack' the difference between an unhealthy negative emotion (disturbance) and a healthy negative emotion (dissatisfaction) by distinguishing between their behavioural and cognitive referents. As an example, Table 7.2 outlines the differences in this respect with respect to

Table 7.2 Behavioural and cognitive referents that help clients to distinguish between anxiety and concern

Adversity	◆ You are facing a threat to your personal domain	
Emotion	**Anxiety**	**Concern**
Behaviour	◆ You avoid the threat ◆ You withdraw physically from the threat ◆ You ward off the threat (e.g. by rituals or superstitious behaviour) ◆ You try to neutralize the threat (e.g. by being nice to people of whom you are afraid) ◆ You distract yourself from the threat by engaging in other activity ◆ You keep checking on the current status of the threat hoping to find that it has disappeared or become benign ◆ You seek reassurance from others that the threat is benign ◆ You seek support from others so that if the threat happens they will handle it or be there to rescue you ◆ You overprepare to minimize the threat happening or so that you are prepared to meet it (NB: It is the overpreparation that is the problem here) ◆ You tranquillize your feelings so that you don't think about the threat ◆ You overcompensate for feeling vulnerable by seeking out an even greater threat to prove to yourself that you can cope	◆ You face up to the threat without using any safety-seeking measures ◆ You take constructive action to deal with the threat ◆ You seek support from others to help you face up to the threat and then take constructive action by yourself rather than rely on them to handle it for you or to be there to rescue you ◆ You prepare to meet the threat but do not overprepare

Table 7.2 Continued

Subsequent thinking	Threat-exaggerated thinking	
	◆ You overestimate the probability of the threat occurring ◆ You underestimate your ability to cope with the threat ◆ You ruminate about the threat ◆ You create an even more negative threat in your mind ◆ You magnify the negative consequences of the threat and minimize its positive consequences ◆ You have more task-irrelevant thoughts than in concern	◆ You are realistic about the probability of the threat occurring ◆ You view the threat realistically ◆ You realistically appraise your ability to cope with the threat ◆ You think about what to do concerning dealing with threat constructively rather than ruminate about the threat ◆ You have more task-relevant thoughts than in anxiety
	Safety-seeking thinking ◆ You withdraw mentally from the threat ◆ You try to persuade yourself that the threat is not imminent and that you are 'imagining' it ◆ You think in ways designed to reassure yourself that the threat is benign or if not, that its consequences will be insignificant ◆ You distract yourself from the threat, for example by focusing on mental scenes of safety and wellbeing ◆ You overprepare mentally to minimize the threat happening or so that you are prepared to meet it (NB. Once again it is the overpreparation that is the problem here) ◆ You picture yourself dealing with the threat in a masterful way ◆ You overcompensate for your feeling of vulnerability by picturing yourself dealing effectively with an even bigger threat	

anxiety and concern. I refer the interested reader to Dryden (2012) for information on the differences between the eight unhealthy negative emotions and their healthy counterparts listed in Table 7.1. The important point to remember here is to encourage clients to consider negotiating healthy negative emotions and their behavioural and cognitive referents as goals in the face of adversity.

Once clients have achieved their 'addressing disturbance' goals and are now healthily dissatisfied about their adversities, they are now ready to set goals that address their dissatisfied psychological state.

Negotiating 'addressing dissatisfaction' goals

In thinking about helping clients to set 'addressing dissatisfaction' goals, it is useful to consider the Serenity prayer attributed to Reinhold Niebuhr: 'God, grant me the serenity to accept the things I cannot change, the courage to change the things I can, and the wisdom to know the difference' (Narcotics Anonymous, 1976). The following are relevant 'addressing dissatisfaction' goals.

Goals that relate to the probable existence of the adversity

In the case example that I gave (see above) the client was anxious about giving an upcoming public presentation to his Board of Directors because he predicted that he would reveal gaps in his knowledge and more importantly that the Directors would consider that he was not up to his job. I called this latter inference an 'adversity' because it was what my client was most anxious about in the situation. Once the client has achieved the dissatisfied psychological state of being concerned rather than being in the disturbed psychological state of being anxious, he is in a position to stand back and consider the accuracy of his prediction. While *how* the therapist does this falls outside of my brief, as it involves considering what therapeutic tasks can be used to achieve such goals, the end result is that the client should be in a position to come to a conclusion on the inference accuracy question. When I am working in this area, I am guided by the idea that the client's judgement is best informed by the concept known in the field of perceptual psychology as the 'best bet' and in philosophy as the 'inference to the best explanation' (Lipton, 2004). Thus, I encourage the client to assume that an inference of adversity is probably true if it provides an explanation of the available data. If not, I encourage him to develop and accept as probably true an alternative inference. Quite often, the client's inference of adversity does not fit the available data and can be rejected and when the client does this, their dissatisfaction disappears because they no longer think that the adversity exists.

Goals that seek to change the adversity (if it can be changed)

If the inference of adversity has been accepted as probably true (e.g. it is probably true that a client's friend is angry with the client), then the client can be helped to set goals that are designed to change the adversity. Care has to be taken here, and there is an important distinction to be made between goals that represent the client's enactment of behaviour designed to bring about change in the adversity that is in the client's control (talking to his friend to help diffuse the friend's anger towards the client) and the change or otherwise itself, which is not in the client's direct control. You should encourage your client to set the former goal rather than the latter.

You should remember that behaviour designed to change an adversity is best carried out when your client is in a dissatisfied psychological state rather than in a disturbed psychological state.

Goals that seek to change the situation in which the adversity occurs (if it can be changed)

Earlier in the chapter I distinguished between an adversity (what your client is most disturbed about in a situation) and the situation in which the adversity occurs. For example, your client has not been invited to a work meeting (actual situation) and infers that this is because he is not liked at work (adversity). Similar considerations should be borne in mind when you come to help your client to set a goal designed to change the situation in which the adversity occurs, if it can be changed, as those when you worked to help your client set a goal designed to change the adversity. Once again, encourage your client to set the enactment of a change-directed behaviour as a goal rather than the effect of that behaviour. Thus, you can encourage your client to approach the person in charge of sending out invitations to the meeting with the purpose of getting an invitation.

Relevant goals when the adversity and/or situation cannot be changed

What can you do when the adversity and/or the situation in which it occurred cannot be changed or your client's efforts to change them have not proven successful. Don't forget, however, that your client is, at this point, in a dissatisfied rather than a disturbed psychological state of mind so if the worst comes to the worst you can help your client to live with the adversity and remain in a dissatisfied psychological state of mind when they cannot help but focus on the situation/adversity. However, you do have other options here. Thus, you can help the client to set the following goals:

◆ to remain in the environment but to avoid the situation/adversity as much as possible;

◆ to change the environment and move away from the situation/adversity as long as this does not impact negatively on your client's life;

◆ to develop mindfulness skills so your client does not dwell on the adversity;

◆ to act in ways consistent with one's values even though the situation/adversity continues to exist.

Negotiating 'promoting development' goals

Once you have helped your client achieve their 'addressing disturbance' goals and their 'addressing dissatisfaction' goals, you are now in a position to help them achieve goals that relate to their growth or development. Mackrill (2011) calls these 'life goals'. These are goals that are designed to help your client get more out of their work, their relationships, and their life in general. The more specific these goals are, the more likely they are to be pursued and thus achieved, although it may that these goals are more likely to be process in nature, that is goals that involve the achievement and continuation of behaviour (e.g. to jog for an hour a day, six days a week) than to involve a definite endpoint. The way the field has developed, it is fair to say that addressing disturbance and dissatisfaction goals are deemed to be largely the province of psychotherapy and counselling (the focus of this text), while promoting development goals is deemed to be largely the province of coaching.

Addressing obstacles to effective goal-negotiation

When negotiating goals it is worth taking your time helping your client to set a realistic goal. In particular, there are a number of obstacles to negotiate while effectively negotiating such a goal and you will need to address these when you identify them. Below some of the most common obstacles are described, along with brief guidelines concerning how to respond if you encounter them in psychotherapy and counselling.

When your client sets a vague goal

Your client may set a vague goal and if so, it is important that you help them to make this goal as specific as possible. Examples of vague goals are: 'I want to be happy', 'I want to get over my anxiety', and 'I want to get on with my life'. A commonly used acronym represents an antidote to vague goals. It is SMART. SMART goals are those that are: specific, measurable, attainable, realistic, and timely. It is useful to remember this acronym when helping clients to set goals that address disturbance and dissatisfaction and those that promote development.

When your client wants to change 'A'

Often your client may wish to change the 'A', either the actual situation and/or the adversity rather than changing their unconstructive responses to the 'A' to those that are constructive. If this is the case and 'A' can be changed, help them to understand that the best chance they have to change 'A' is when they are in a healthy frame of mind to do so and this is achieved when their responses to this 'A' are constructive. So before they can change 'A', they need to change their disturbed responses at 'C'.

When your client wants to change another person

When your client's target problem is centred on their relationship to another person or group of people, then their goal may be to change the other(s). You need to help your client to see that this goal is inappropriate as others' behaviour is not under the direct control of your client. However, attempts to influence others are under your client's direct control and *may* lead to such behavioural change. As such, they are appropriate goals. In such cases, however, it is often important to help the client consider their responses when their influence attempts do not work. Helping clients to deal constructively with such failed attempts is often important in such cases. And of course, don't forget that the best time for your client to influence another person for the better is when they are in a dissatisfied and not in a disturbed frame of mind. Thus, if your client is in a disturbed frame of mind and wishes to change another person, you are faced with two tasks. First, you need to provide your client with an acceptable rationale for negotiating an 'addressing disturbance' goal, and then you need to help him understand that it is important to set a goal that is within his control (i.e. his behaviour) rather than the outcome of his behaviour (which is outside his control).

When your client sets a goal based on experiencing less of the problematic response

Often when asked about their goals in relation to the adversity at 'A', clients say that want to feel less of the disturbed emotion that is featured in their target problem (e.g. less anxious). While many therapists may accept this as a legitimate goal, I do not for the following reason. REBT theory which underpins my approach to goal negotiation argues when a client holds a rigid belief they take a preference (e.g. for acceptance) and turn it into a rigid belief (e.g. 'I want to be accepted, and therefore I have to be'). When they hold a flexible belief they take the same preference and keep it flexible by negating possible rigidity (e.g. I want to be accepted, but it is not necessary that I am). In both the rigid belief and the flexible belief the strength of the unhealthy negative emotion in the first case and of the healthy negative emotion in the second is determined by the strength of the preference when that preference is not met. The stronger the preference under these circumstances the stronger the negative emotion of both types. Based on this analysis, my goal is to help the person experience a healthy negative emotion of relative intensity to the unhealthy negative emotion rather than to encourage them to strive to experience an unhealthy negative emotion of decreased intensity.

When your client sets a goal based on experiencing the absence of the problematic response

You also need to be prepared when your client nominates the absence of the problem as their goal (e.g. 'I don't want to feel anxious when giving a talk'). When your client says this, it is important to help them see that it is not possible to live in a response vacuum and from there you can discuss the presence of a set of healthy responses to their adversity as their goal.

When your client sets as a goal a positive response to the actual situation and bypasses the adversity

Another situation that may well occur when you ask a client for their goal is that they may nominate a positive response to the actual situation while bypassing the adversity. For example, if my client in the case example had taken this tack he would have said something like, 'I want to become confident at giving public presentations'. In doing so he would have bypassed his dealing with adversity, which was revealing gaps in his knowledge and being thought of as not up to doing his job. A good response to this client would be to ask him how he could become confident at giving public presentations as long as he was anxious about being judged negatively by his Board of Directors. By helping this client to deal with this issue first and set an appropriate goal with respect to his adversity, I would be helping him to take the next step and work towards increasing his confidence about his performance. Taking this approach is akin to a situation where your client wants to get to Windsor (confidence) from London (anxiety) by train, but the only way of doing so is to get to Slough (concern) and change trains there to Windsor (confidence), as there is no direct train from London (anxiety) to Windsor (confidence). Figure 7.1 depicts these two routes.

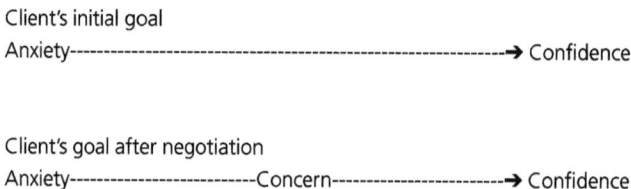

Client's initial goal
Anxiety---→ Confidence

Client's goal after negotiation
Anxiety---------------------------Concern------------------------→ Confidence

Fig. 7.1 Two routes to confidence.

When a client wants to feel indifferent in the face of an adversity

Sometimes a client says that their goal is not to care about a particular adversity when, in reality, they do care about it. Indeed, their disturbed feelings indicate that they do care. My practice is to help my client understand what not caring or indifference means as follows:

WD: Now Albion Rovers are playing Brechin City on Saturday in the Scottish 1st Division. Do you care who wins?

CLIENT: Not at all.

WD: That is what not caring means. Faced with a choice between two options you can't choose between them because you literally don't care what happens. Now when you say you want not to care if you get promoted do you mean that faced with the choice of getting promoted or not getting promoted you want me to help you to be indifferent about the outcome?

CLIENT: I guess not.

WD: Because would you prefer to be promoted or not to be promoted.

CLIENT: To be promoted.

WD: So rather than not care if you don't get promoted, how about if I help you to care about it but not to be disturbed about it should it happen?

CLIENT: Yes, that make sense.

I then helped the client to understand what the behavioural and cognitive referents of non-disturbed caring would be so that he could strive for this psychological state.

When a client nominates a goal that is dangerous or unrealistic

Sometimes a client nominates a goal that is in Law & Jacob's (2015) terms 'unacceptable'. What they mean is that the goal is either 'dangerous (e.g. a person with anorexia wanting to set a goal to lose weight, or someone with depression wanting to be helped to end their life), or because a goal is unrealistic (e.g. someone with a physical disability wanting to be a professional footballer)' (Law & Jacob, 2015: 16). As Law & Jacob (2015) go on to say, these goals should not be dismissed, but should be a prelude for discussion and careful re-negotiation. Helping the client to imagine responding to a friend who nominates such goals can be particularly helpful here in providing the client with sufficient distance to enable them to participate in their own goal re-negotiation with the therapist.

The importance of negotiating goals based on values

As a therapist, you will be aware of the limited time that you have with your clients, particularly if you work within a brief therapy framework and therefore you need to discover ways of increasing the chances that what clients achieve from the process endures. One way of doing this is to help the client to find an important value that might underpin their goal, as goals that are under-pinned by values are more likely to be achieved than goals that aren't (Eccles & Wigfield, 2002).

Case example

In my work with another client, I discovered that one of his stated core values was honesty. In negotiating an 'addressing disturbance' about something that he regarded as a defect, I helped him to set a goal of feeling disappointed about having the defect rather than ashamed about it. Then, having helped him to achieve this healthy negative emotional goal, he was then faced with a choice of whether to choose to show what he regarded as a defect or hide it, as he was sure others would notice it and scorn him for it. His core value of honesty led him to choose to show it while feeling disappointed but not ashamed, rather than hide it. After he did so, he realized that others either did not notice his so-called defect or complimented him on his courage for showing it.

Points for reflection

- If a client nominated a goal of indifference in the face of an adversity, how would you respond?
- What is your view on the issue of clients wanting to feel less anxious in the face of threat?
- What core values do you have as a person that would have a positive influence on your goal-setting in an area where you wish to make a change?
- In your opinion as a therapist, what makes for a 'good' goal?

Further reading

Dryden, W. (2012). *Dealing with emotional problems using rational—emotive cognitive behaviour therapy: A practitioner's guide.* Hove, East Sussex: Routledge.
A text which clearly outlines the eight major problematic emotions for which people seek therapeutic help and their healthy negative emotional alternatives. Each healthy and unhealthy negative emotion is distinguished by associated behaviour and thinking. This information helps therapists encourage their clients to set healthy negative responses to adversity as 'addressing disturbance' goals.

Law. D., & Jacob. J. (2015). *Goals and goal based outcomes (GBOs): Some useful information. 3rd edition.* London: CAMHS Press.

A clearly written booklet on therapeutic goals and goal-based outcomes that will be useful for therapists from a range of orientations.

Mackrill, T. (2011) Differentiating life goals and therapeutic goals: Expanding our understanding of the working alliance. *British Journal of Guidance & Counselling, 39*, 25–39.

This paper makes an important distinction between clients' life goals and their therapy goals. The paper explores five problematic life goals and how therapy goals may help to address them.

Mahrer, A. (Ed.). (1967). *The goals of psychotherapy.* New York: Appleton-Century.

This is a classic text on the subject of goals in therapy and clearly shows that experts consider that therapy is designed not only to address issues of psychological disturbance, but also to promote growth or development.

References

Dryden, W. (2012). *Dealing with emotional problems using rational—emotive cognitive behaviour therapy: A practitioner's guide.* Hove, East Sussex: Routledge.

Eccles, J.S., & Wigfield, A. (2002). Motivational beliefs, values and goals. *Annual Review of Psychology, 53*, 109–32.

Law. D., & Jacob. J. (2015). *Goals and goal based outcomes (GBOs): Some useful information. 3rd edition.* London: CAMHS Press.

Lipton, P. (2004). *Inference to the best explanation. 2nd edition.* Abingdon, Oxon: Routledge.

Mackrill, T. (2011) Differentiating life goals and therapeutic goals: Expanding our understanding of the working alliance. *British Journal of Guidance & Counselling, 39*, 25–39.

Mahrer, A. (Ed.). (1967). *The goals of psychotherapy.* New York: Appleton-Century.

Narcotics Anonymous (1976). *NA white booklet.* Chatsworth, CA: Narcotics Anonymous World Services, Inc.

Chapter 8

Goal-oriented practice

Duncan Law

This chapter will focus on the application of goals and goal-setting in goal-oriented therapeutic practice. It will:

◆ set the clinical context for goal-oriented practice;

◆ explore ideas around goal-setting and using goals in practice;

◆ set out how service systems and structures can support goal-oriented practice;

◆ look at the goal-oriented practice in supervision and consultation.

Case examples and transcripts are offered throughout the chapter not as examples of perfect practice (I never feel we learn much as therapists from snippets of others' moments of therapeutic perfection), but are presented to illustrate goal-oriented practice in action. The examples are based on real case scenarios but for the sake of anonymity and to create succinct case examples that are relevant to this chapter, some details have been changed and merged.

Goal-oriented practice

Over recent years there has been a shift in the focus of therapy and mental health in general away from the medical, diagnostic questions: 'What's wrong with you?' to the more collaborative, formulation-driven question: 'What's happened to you?' (Division of Clinical Psychology, 2011). This chapter argues that the starting point of any intervention and the primary focus of therapy should be: 'What do you want to change?'. 'What do you want to change?', invites the client to share their hopes and wishes for the outcome of a therapeutic encounter: what they want to be different as a result of the effort and what resource they will need to invest in the therapy—in short it asks for an expression of the client's 'goals'.

This shift to goal-oriented practice necessarily includes the need to understand the 'problem' through diagnosis or formulation, but it emphasizes the primary purpose of therapy from being one of 'understanding' to being one of 'change'. This is not to play down the power of understanding as an intervention in creating shift, but in goal-oriented practice the emphasis is on the client's wish for change and the therapy and therapist is guided by, and focused on, the change goal: 'what I want to be different'.

In this sense goal-oriented practice is a therapeutic stance rather than a therapeutic model. Once a therapy goal has been collaboratively agreed it is possible to use any suitable intervention to reach it. Goal-oriented practice does not dictate any particular therapeutic model in which to reach the goal, but rather provides a focus, or a direction of travel, that the therapist and client have *agreed* to work on together to reach. It works on the pluralistic principle that there are many potential vehicles that can take you towards the same destination (Cooper and McLeod, 2011). However, we need to be careful not to fall down the postmodernist, constructionist, black hole of 'anything goes'. Research shows us that some vehicles—therapeutic interventions—are more likely to get you to where you want to be than others, and indeed some vehicles may not get you there at all (Roth & Fonagy 2013).

Goal-oriented practice is simply any therapeutic encounter that works towards helping the person, be it an adult, young person, child, family, or community, move towards what they want to get out of the endeavour of a therapeutic intervention. A 'goal' is simply a shorthand for 'what I want to be different if therapy is successful'. Whatever phrase we choose to name 'goals', it is the concept behind the phrase: 'goal-oriented practice', that is of importance here.

It might be argued that this is no different in purpose from pretty much all therapy. That is, even the most non-directive and exploratory of therapy models have implicit goals; something along the lines of 'I want to understand myself better' or 'I want to experience this process'. In anything we choose to take part in, we have to take an active role. Therapy has to be active (even if it means actively remaining silent or actively not turning up) and anything active is goal-oriented, even if we have not voiced it, or even if we are not consciously aware of it. The difference with goal-oriented practice is the degree to which the goals are made explicit, collaboratively agreed, perceived as jointly owned, and form a focus for change—rather than implicit, and separately or just therapist-owned goals. In goal-oriented practice the goals of the client and the goals of the therapist are made explicit, and the therapy takes place where these goals overlap, are co-constructed and collaboratively agreed.

Setting therapy goals

The activity of therapy requires motivation to sustain it (Holtforth & Michalak 2012). Therapy is an active process with costs attached: the time taken out of a busy life to attend sessions, or the emotional resource needed to sustain what is often a difficult and challenging process. Even the very young who are brought to therapy by parents or carers, or those incarcerated in institutions with therapy orders placed on them, or parents involved with the social care system around safeguarding concerns, all still have to be motivated to engage, or disengage, with the proscribed intervention. The 'what do I want to be different from this encounter' (the goal), balanced with the other side of the equation 'is it worth the effort' (the perceived cost of reaching the goal) provide the sum of the motivation. For therapy to be sustained, motivation needs to be sustained and goal-oriented practice can help provide a focus and clarity about motivation at the start of an intervention. This focus on a shared goal strengthens the therapeutic alliance (Bordin 1979) and increases motivation.

Case example: using goals to focus motivation

Making therapy goals explicit can help make the motivation explicit. As we have stated, for most, therapy is a choice, but for some it is an imposition. How do we collaborate to construct therapy goals when the 'client' is not a client by choice? How can goal-oriented practice help find a motivational focus for the therapy?

Bob was a 39-year-old man with convictions for violence—he had been referred for therapy as part of his probation order but he was a reluctant client; angry at the criminal justice system and angry at the thought of seeing a therapist. The initial couple of sessions were filled with his rage at a process that he secretly felt (which he shared later) would 'get inside my head'. He feared being a passive underdog in therapy controlled by another person, which caused him understandable anxiety given his life experiences growing up—lack of power meant lack of control which, in turn, led to violence. The therapist was keen to move the focus of the session from: 'I'm here because I have to be', to 'I'm here because there may be something I can get from it'. Using variations of the solution-focused therapy 'miracle questions' (de Shazer, 1991) can be really helpful here. After a great deal of preliminary discussion the therapist asked:

THERAPIST: I know you really don't want to come here and I know you really don't feel you need to be here—but let's just suppose for a moment that this might be helpful even in some small way—if we can look back after three months say and despite all your doubts something surprising had happened and something had changed and even in a small way it had been helpful— what would you want that change to have been?

BOB: I'd have got rid of the probation officer.

THERAPIST: Got rid?

BOB: Yeah, he'd be gone, out of my life… stop hassling me.

THERAPIST: So the probation officer would be out of your life—or at least not hassling you—or not hassle you as much perhaps?

Here the therapist is trying to shape the initial wish of Bob: to be rid of the probation officer all together, into a goal that was realistic in the medium term. The probation period meant the probation officer would not be 'gone' completely but he might be less 'hassle'.

BOB: Yeah.

THERAPIST: We can work on that …

BOB: What!

THERAPIST: We can work on that together—to get the probation officer off your back quite so much as he is now… If after three months the probation officer were hassling you less—is that something worth working on together?

BOB: Yeah.

This 'goal', 'to reduce the amount of hassle from the probation officer', is not the most therapeutic of goals—it is not an 'approach goal', nor a particularly 'high order goal' (see Chapter 3, this volume). As practitioners we sometimes have to go with goals that are good enough and remain pragmatic to the possibilities of the therapeutic context. 'Therapy orders' are never a good context for collaborative practice, but for Bob it provided him some internal motivation to attend and for the therapist and Bob together it gave a focus for the sessions: 'what would have to change to get the probation officer to be less hassle'. In this case it opened up discussions of violence as a way of feeling 'safe'. The therapist and client explored the dilemma, on the one hand, of violence and aggression keeping the probation officer worried and therefore more 'hassle', with Bob feeling more in control. Or, on the other hand, Bob being calmer and less aggressive (but risking feeling vulnerable) and reducing the anxiety of the officer and chancing a reduction of the hassle. This intervention provided no great 'cure'. Bob's difficulties, of layer upon layer of trauma, were beyond what could be achieved in a six-month treatment order. However, it did open up some space for Bob to think about his impact on others and provide space to begin to mentalize (Bateman & Fonagy, 2012). The hope was that it opened the door for further conversations for Bob, ideally with a trusted person in a trusted environment—not because of a therapy order with a stranger.

Case example: negotiating safe goals

In the previous example the goal-setting task was to find common ground on what kind of goals could be chosen to work on in therapy. In some cases the task is to find any overlap at all between the client's goals and what is safe and acceptable to work on in the context of therapy.

Jo was a 13-year-old girl referred to a child mental health service with concerns about her low weight—her parents disclosed their concerns that she had been losing weight over the past six months, her periods had stopped, and she was exercising to what they considered excess, while at the same time restricting her food intake. In the first part of the session, Jo's parents had shared their worries and discussed their goals: 'to get our little girl back and to see her happy and eating again'. In the second part of the session, the therapist met with Jo on her own to give her a chance to talk about her concerns away from the understandable anxiety of her parents. Initially in the tentative exploration of what Jo wanted (having heard her parents express their goals and wishes), she spoke of how she wanted 'to lose weight—another half a stone'. This goal was clearly not safe but not at all unusual with young people's issues around body image—the task of the therapist was to try and find some overlap between the goals that Jo held and those that would be safe to agree to work on together. After some discussion to understand Jo's feelings behind the goals and to explore the Jo's ideas around losing weight and her parents' views, the therapist saw their task as being to work with Jo to find safe goals acceptable to both that they could work on together. The therapist began by exploring potential safer goals that might be hidden behind the initial unsafe goal:

THERAPIST: So, Jo, you have been really clear that what you would really like is to lose more weight—half a stone? Is that right?

JO: Yes—I feel fat—people stare at me because of that, particularly in PE ... I feel fat, and unhappy, I don't have any friends. .....

THERAPIST: That sounds really uncomfortable ... feeling that people are staring at you. ..... Let's just think for a moment about what you hope life would be like if you lost half a stone? How do you think things would be different?

JO: I wouldn't be fat.

THERAPIST: OK, what else would be different?

JO: If I wasn't so fat I'd feel happier, and more confident.

THERAPIST: ... and if you were feeling happier and more confident ... ?

JO: I'd probably have more friends too.

THERAPIST: So if you lost half a stone; you might feel more confident, feel happier, and start to have more friends?

JO: Yes—I think so. ....

At this point the therapist is starting to get a glimpse of Jo's safer goals behind the unsafe one of losing half a stone: 'to feel happy, more confident, and have more friends'. This opens up the possibility of exploring these higher-order goals further, and might, over time, lead to forming agreed goals that the therapist, Jo, and her parents can agree to work on. In Jo's case this took another few sessions. This was, in part, because of her firm commitment that the only thing that could help would be to lose more weight and further hindered by the necessity to start a re-feeding plan. Both of these factors had a big negative impact on the therapeutic relationship.

'Vehicles' and 'destinations'

Sometimes when clients state their goals they are stating goals that are a vehicle to get to a goal rather than a destination goal: somewhere they want to arrive. If we take this travel analogy a step further—end goals or 'destination' goals can be seen as where in the world you want to get to eventually: 'New York' or 'somewhere hot with a beach', or 'anywhere but here'. Vehicle goals are what you need to do to get to your destination: 'fly', 'take a train', 'walk'. Part of the task of setting goals is to make sure the task alliance is around a destination goal and not just the vehicle goal. Other examples of vehicle goals are 'I want my child to be diagnosed with ADHD' or 'I want psychotherapy' or 'I want to get married'— the question to ask, when presented with a vehicle is ' … and what do you hope will be different if you get: the diagnosis/psychotherapy/married?', to which the answers might be: 'I will understand my child better and can be a better parent/ I'll be contented with who I am/I'll be happy'.

In Jo's case her vehicle was '*to lose more weight*'. The therapy task at this stage was to understand her destination goals: where her vehicle of 'losing more weight' would get her. After the conversation in which Jo and the therapist discovered that Jo felt insecure and unhappy and she felt that losing weight was the way to feel 'more confident and be happy and have friends'—this was her destination goal or higher order goal (see Chapter 3, this volume, for further discussion of goal hierarchies).

It is important to avoid therapy traps of setting goals that are vehicles and not destinations. Otherwise we may end up working with apparent goals that may be, at worst, dangerous for the client or, at best, just a statement of a process for reaching a goal but not a goal in itself. By reflecting on whether a stated goal really is a therapy goal that can be worked on collaboratively, we are more likely to build a working alliance with the client and achieve a better outcome.

Goal-oriented practice, shared-decision making, and intervention planning

Once the goal is clearly defined it is important to establish and agree how best to get there (the vehicle)—if this is not already clear. For some this may mean a discussion about whether the client's preferred mode of transport will actually get them there (will losing weight really lead to increased confidence and happiness?). This might mean a conversation (which may be a long and complex conversation) looking for alternatives that may be more appropriate to the task. Further conversation around what, and who else, might help make the change can be established. Therapy by itself is never the whole answer to psychological difficulties; indeed the evidence suggests that for some it is no answer at all (Wolpert, 2016).

In the previous examples the therapist had be more directive than usual to try and reach an agreed goal for therapy. For most people therapy is a choice to participate. In such cases there is more opportunity to co-construct and collaboratively agree goals. This approach is not only a more transparent and ethical approach, but also a common factor of evidence-based practice. Collaborating to reach shared and agreed goals with the client is a vital step in development of a good therapeutic alliance, which is one of the best predictors of clinical outcomes (Horvath *et al.*, 2011).

The process of shared decision making (SDM) is a method to aid collaborative goal-setting, which is particularly helpful when choosing intervention options. The concept of SDM has evolved from physical health settings where recognition was given that patients were experts in their own lives and bodies, and treatment decisions were more effective if the medical practitioner and the patient made decisions together about intervention plans (Edwards & Elwyn, 2009). The same process is known to be true in psychological practice (Tryon & Winograd, 2011, see Chapter 5, this volume). The stance of SDM is to set out the problem and be clear about the boundaries in which the decision is taking place, what are the intervention options, and what are the pros and cons of each option.

Despite evidence of the positive impact on therapy outcomes from collaborative goal-setting and intervention planning (Orlinsky Rønnestad & Willutzki 2004), they are not always prominent features of therapeutic practice. In part, this is because of the complex nature of people and psychological problems, and the contexts in which they exist. As we have seen it is often difficult to collaborate to set goals and intervention plans, despite best efforts. However, the lack of collaborative goal-oriented practice is also a result of some hard-to-shift elements of therapy culture. It still greatly disappoints me to hear clients tell stories of clinicians with whom they have met, whose formulations consist of (to paraphrase only a little) 'there seems to be a problem' and whose treatment plan consists of, 'let's keep meeting until the problem is gone'. Such a vague and unfocused approach to therapy is not only unhelpful, it runs counter to evidence-based practice. Moreover, it is also unethical as it negates any chance of informed consent to treatment.

For consent to treatment to be 'informed', the client must be given all of the information about what the treatment involves: what the expected outcomes might be, including risks, what reasonable alternative treatments are available, and the consequences of not having the treatment (Department of Health, 2009). Without the focus for therapy that goals bring and without the associated intervention plan to reach the goal, consent cannot be informed and this raises both ethical and legal issues. As therapists we should be interested in legal and ethical issues not through fear of litigation or disciplinary proceedings with our respective professional bodies but because the ethical and legal issues are based on what is in the client's best interest—and this should be at the forefront of all we do. This leads not only to ethical practice but to effective practice. Goal-oriented practice, derived through a process of SDM; with its explicit expression of goals and intervention planning to reach those goals, facilitates informed consent.

Formulations and goal-oriented practice

Shared formulations are where the therapist and client co-create a story or narrative that describes and explains the issues the person wants help with. Formulations make sense of the social, psychological, and biological context in which the problem exists ('What has happened to you?'), link the problem to the goal ('What do you want to change?' or 'Where do you want to get to?'), and give pointers to the possible ways to reach the goal (the vehicles to get to the destination). Good formulations link these components in ways that are coherent and logical to both therapist and client, and explain how the intervention might help reach the goal. Simple structures can aid the development of shared and coherent formulations. In turn these can help in the application of goal-oriented and evidence-informed practice, and informed consent, by providing clear links among:

- the client's goals;
- the activity expected to be helpful in reaching those goals;
- why that activity should help (the logic);
- clarity about how progress towards the goal can be monitored (to check the therapy is making the expected difference).

Case example: an older lady with anxiety

Mary was a 67-year-old woman who had suffered with anxiety for some years. Her goal was to feel less anxious so she could get on with her life. During the assessment it became clear that Mary had begun avoiding places and situations in which she had felt anxious, and this avoidance had spread to the point where she had become virtually housebound. Table 8.1 shows how the application of this approach can help both the therapist and the client develop a coherent formulation and recognize the links among goals, the model of therapy being offered, and the expected outcomes; thereby offering clarity on how the intervention might help and how best to monitor change towards her goals.

Goal-oriented systems and settings

A therapist's adoption of a goal-oriented approach is largely one of choice (and of course their own higher order goals as to what kind of therapist they want to be). But there are also systems and settings that can encourage and support the adopting of this stance—particularly helpful where a therapist might work in multidisciplinary team settings.

Table 8.1 Process/logic model for reaching Mary's goals

Process/logic model components [How they were applied for Mary's difficulties]	Therapy components
What is the outcome goal? [Collaboratively agreed goals between Mary and her therapist]	To feel less anxious
What are the contributing factors? [Based on the information gathered in the assessment from the development of the shared formulation]	Avoidance of perceived anxiety-provoking situations, anxious thinking style, lack of social network
What change mechanism might help? [Linked to the formulation]	Exposure to anxiety and help to change thinking styles to help control and challenge anxious thoughts better
What is the activity needed? [Based on the evidence base that fits best with Mary's goals and wishes]	Group cognitive behavioural therapy (CBT) to help with thinking styles and manage exposure
What is the resource needed? [Based on the evidence of effectiveness for this kind of intervention]	Attend weekly 50-minutes sessions for approximately 12 weeks
Expected (measurable) short-term outcomes [Measure that best fits with the expected outcomes and is acceptable to Mary]	Self-rating on a goal-based outcome measure, progress to goal of feeling less anxious (and consider the use of a standardized anxiety symptom measure)
Expected longer-term outcomes [Derived from Mary's higher order life goals]	Living a more fulfilled life, not restricted by fear and anxiety

Example: goal-oriented systems: the Choice and Partnership Approach (CAPA)

There are service models that place goal-oriented practice at the heart of the delivery system, and not just at the heart of the therapy. The Choice and Partnership Approach (CAPA) (York and Kingsbury, 2013) is a clinical system that grew out of child mental health services in the UK. The model brings together ideas from 'lean thinking' (making sure limited resources are used as effectively as possible by avoiding waste). CAPA combines these ideas with 'demand and capacity modelling' (ensuring resources are deployed in the most effective way to ensure services or clinics have the capacity (enough therapists) to meet the demands on the service (the people needing the service)).

CAPA conceptualizes therapeutic encounters into two parts. The first is *choice*: working collaboratively with the client to identify what they want to change; and *partnership*: working together to make those changes. The task of the 'choice' part of the encounter is: 'to find out what they want to be different, discuss different ways of achieving this goal and then ensuring they are seen by someone best suited to help them' (York and Kingsbury, 2013, p. 64). Central to the model is the idea of matching the client to the right therapist and to the therapy model that is most likely to meet the goals and wishes of the client. Note that, however skilled a therapist is and however wide a skill set of interventions they have to draw upon, no one has all the skills and knowledge necessary to help every client reach all their goals. This challenges the belief that certain therapy modalities are the panacea for mental distress. It is not always necessary to pass on clients to other colleagues to do the work if the therapist, him or herself, has the skills to meet the goals of the client. However, the added benefit of a change in therapist for partnership is that it encourages clear goal-setting at the choice appointment, which leads to more defined and focused intervention plans. To match goal to therapist, both therapist and client must have agreed goals at the start of the intervention process (the choice point). For most clients, therapy goals can be collaboratively agreed relatively quickly; enough, at least, to decide on the broad interventions most likely to be effective in the 'partnership' phase of the work. The model allows for the likelihood that these broad therapy goals require further refinement in the early stages of therapy. For a minority, however, and particularly in settings in which the mental health issues are less acute or less severe, clients may struggle to identify therapy goals. In these cases the goal may be more exploratory: 'to discover what I want from life' or 'to see if I can understand what's bothering me'. In these examples the goals are to 'discover' and 'understand'. In a sense they are meta-goals (Chapter 3, this volume): goals to find goals, but they are goals nonetheless.

Either way, only once a goal has been agreed and some discussion has taken place about the possible vehicles (modalities) to reach the goal, matches can be made among the client and their goals and the intervention and the best therapist to provide this intervention. The matching process puts pressure on the therapists in the system to develop clear goals and interventions plans with the client before embarking on an intervention. This ensures the intervention (and therapist) are likely to be a good match and therefore leads to efficient and effective deployment of resources. For the client with more exploratory goals to 'discover' or 'understand', the intervention and therapist must be matched to provide this exploratory space. For the client with more focused goals, the match can be more attuned to a therapist who has the skills to provide an evidence-based intervention that fits with these goals.

Case example: the two Jacks: same problems, same goals, different interventions

How a goal is reached is dependent on the unique context of the client and their choices about how to reach goals. The same goals (destination), even if attached to the same problem might still lead to different interventions (vehicles) for getting there, as we can see here in these two examples.

The two Jacks were unrelated 13-year-old boys who for the last two years had suffered with anxiety that was preventing them from being in school. Both boys had identical goals of 'getting back into school'. During the choice appointment with the first Jack, it was revealed that his difficulties had begun when he moved to secondary school aged 11 years. He had always struggled in school academically, he struggled to read and write, and analysis of his early development revealed he had also walked and talked late. Jack spoke of how much he liked being with his friends at school. He loved football but 'hated the teachers' and often had panic attacks when asked questions in class. After some discussion, the therapist shared with Jack and his parents their tentative formulation of the difficulties. The therapist spent time slowly and sensitively sharing their thoughts that Jack may have a learning difficulty that had not yet been picked up in school. This might fit with why Jack was experiencing more and more feelings of failure when faced with yet another task that he was unable to achieve, thus leading to the anxiety and panic. They discussed the various options together: that an assessment of Jack's cognitive abilities could be arranged to test out the hypothesis of the learning disability or offer some talking therapy to help Jack manage his anxiety better—all agreed the former was the preferred option. The assessment was arranged that indeed revealed a learning disability. This was shared with the school who was able to put in additional help and Jack got back into school and got on with his life without any need for counselling or psychological therapy.

The second Jack presented with the same difficulty and the same goal: to get back into school—he also had suffered panic attacks for the last two years. In his choice appointment, it became clear that his panics stemmed from an incident in school where Jack had contracted a virus that led to him vomiting. He remembered being jeered at by other school children and the trauma of the event stayed with him long after he was physically better. Although he managed to get back into school after the illness, he was left with anxiety about getting sick again and re-experiencing the shame and isolation he felt on the day he got ill. He had initially started to avoid other children who appeared unwell but, over time, this led him to over-worry about the prospect of being 'contaminated' by contact with other children. Consequently, he had begun to have panic attacks in school and eventually stopped attending altogether. In this scenario it was felt that the triggers for the anxiety were connected to the thoughts of the original incident and compounded by further fears of contamination and the consequent avoidance that kept these fears in place. It was these anxiety thoughts and the remembered trauma that kept this Jack from his goal of getting back into school. Drawing on the evidence base, the therapist discussed with Jack and his parents the idea of working in a cognitive behavioural therapy (CBT) model to tackle the symptoms of trauma and panic. The choice therapist introduced Jack and his family to a CBT specialist colleague to do the partnership work.

In these examples we see that a goal does not dictate the intervention method. As therapists we must always ensure that the interventions fit with both the goal and the unique context of the client.

Using goals to keep focus

Once goals have been collaboratively agreed it is possible to use tools that track progress towards the goal (Law & Bradley, 2013). The usefulness of tracking progress in therapy has been well documented elsewhere (Lambert, 2005; Bickman *et al.*, 2011; Chapter 6, this volume). If used well, clinically embedded in the therapy, tracking goal progress can provide a measure of clinical outcomes (Wolpert *et al.*, 2012), and facilitate more focused interventions. Without clear therapy goals, the work can become unfocused and both the client and the therapist can become unclear about what the joint venture is in which they are engaged. Here, the therapeutic alliance is weakened and the work may take longer and be less effective (see Chapter 5, this volume).

Colleagues in the USA have devised a standardized tool to identify the client's 'top problems' to be worked on (Weisz *et al.*, 2011). Once the top problems have been identified, the therapist and client agree which are the priorities and these become the focus (goals) of the work. These goals focus the intervention and avoid drift into areas that are distractions from the focus of the approach.

Particular attention is given to dealing with 'crisis of the week' (COW) (Cohen, Berliner, & Mannarino, 2010) that may swamp or overwhelm the family and the therapist. COWs are attended to by listening to the crisis and then linking it back to the agreed goals of the therapy:

> Therapist: "So how would you like to handle this today? We can just talk about it for a few minutes and then get back to our plan for today, or we can use this situation to see if there is any way you would apply what you have been learning. For example, how did you handle the feelings you had about it? How could you use the cognitive triangle to make sense of your reaction and maybe identify some ways to think about it differently? What would you like to do?"
>
> (Cohen, Berliner, & Mannarino, 2010: 222)

The MATCH-ADTC model (Chorpita & Weisz, 2009) is a goal-oriented, modularized method for applying manualized CBT to anxiety depression, trauma, and conduct problems in children and young people. The application of the modularized sessions is flexibly focused around the family's goals.

Conversations around lack of progress towards a goal

In some cases, the therapy process may not run smoothly. Progress may be intermittent and non-linear, with no steady improvement session-by-session. For some there will be little or no progress or progress will be in the opposite direction from that which is hoped for or expected. In these cases, goal-oriented practice can help facilitate conversations around the lack of progress that might lead to changes and improvements in the therapy to better facilitate change. Four interconnected and complementary areas are helpful to consider: the external context, the therapeutic alliance, the therapeutic modality, and the client's own readiness for change.

The biggest influence on change in any person's life is the context in which they live for the 167 hours a week they are not in therapy: relationships, financial issues, family problems, neighbourhood, work, school (Bohart, & Tallman, 2010). Therapy may have the potential to help nudge things in a more helpful direction. This nudge might, over time, lead to a life-altering trajectory for the client, but we should not overemphasize the impact an hour a week of therapy really has in the context of a person's whole life. As such it is just as important to understand the external context of a client as it is to understand the internal context of therapy when understanding progress or lack of progress. We must, however, be careful not to fall into the attribution bias trap of assuming positive therapeutic change is down to our good work and lack of change is down to the client and/or their context.

In goal-oriented practice when reviewing goal progress it is important to explore a range of internal and external factors to help begin to understand a lack of goal progress—these might include:

1. External contextual issues: 'Has anything particular happened this week that might have had an impact on how things have been ... at home, work etc.'

2. The therapeutic alliance: 'Is there anything that we could do differently in this session which might help things move forward? Is there anything I could do that might make things more helpful?' This could also include questions about the goals themselves: 'Do the goals we set at the beginning of the intervention still feel the right ones that you want to work towards?' (Law & Bradley, 2013).

3. The model of therapy: 'Does the way we have been working still seem to be helpful—or do you have some thoughts on what might be a more useful way of doing things?'.

4. The client's readiness to change: 'Do you feel able to make this change at the moment?' or 'Is now the right time to make the changes you want?'.

Clearly the phrasing of the questions would be adapted to fit the client and based on the clinical judgement of the therapist, but it is always helpful to keep these four broad areas in mind.

Using goals to plan endings

There is a commonly held myth in therapy that all people with mental health issues and emotional distress can be helped to the point of recovery ('cured') if only enough time and resource is given to them (Wolpert, 2016). This often translates to clients being offered more and more interventions with more and more intensity. There is scant evidence to support this myth. The most recent evidence from real-world therapy settings in England suggests recovery rates of between 33% in children's services (Wolpert *et al.*, 2016) to around 46% in adult psychological therapy services (NHS Digital, 2016). What this means is that most clients we see are likely not to have recovered at the end of an intervention, however skilled we are, and however hard we try. Yet despite this, many clinicians find it difficult to discuss endings with clients unless things are 'better'. The reality is that clients drop out long before clinicians stop offering appointments.

We need to move to practice that acknowledges this reality and ensures honest collaborative discussions with clients about endings. This is not only at the point of recovery but when either enough progress has been made or when no further progress is expected. Goal-oriented practice can help with these discussions particularly where goals have been tracked. The discussion about endings must start at the beginning—when goals are being agreed and baseline scores are being set. At this point it is important to set the expectation of ending when things are 'good enough' rather than 'perfect'. Conversations around ending should start here:

THERAPIST: So at the moment you rate progress to your goal at one out of ten—what rating do you think things will need to be at before you feel you are back on track enough for us to stop meeting?

or

THERAPIST: we will plan to work together for as long as it seems helpful—not until things are completely ten-out-of-ten. It would be great if you got there, but most people make enough progress towards a goal to feel things are on the right track enough to carry on without the need for further therapy. For some this might be five-out-of-ten, or six-out-of-ten etc.—but we will talk again about this and decide together when this work has gone as far as it is helpful.

In goal-oriented practice, the ending should always be part of the conversation around whether enough progress has been made and using the therapy goals to weigh up the pros and cons of further sessions.

Goal-oriented practice in supervision and consultation

Supervisors have a particularly helpful role to play in helping therapists keep a goal focus and perspective on their therapeutic work and to avoid attribution bias around change (Milne, 2009) Teams that adopt goal-oriented supervision, be it individual or peer supervision, help clinicians keep goal-focused. The CAPA model argues that one of the most important questions a supervisor can ask is 'what are the client's goals?' (York & Kingsbury, 2013). Where cases have drifted, it is often that the therapist has not set collaboratively agreed goals with the client or the work has drifted from these goals. Asking about goals: 'Are there any? Are they still relevant? Are they realistic and achievable? Is the therapeutic intervention the most helpful way to reach these goals?, are simple and effective questions for supervisors to ask to help a therapist think about how focused or otherwise an intervention might have become. Peer supervision also helps make team practice more transparent, and further can help embed a culture of goal-oriented practice across a team.

Case example: goal-oriented supervision

Helping the supervisee reflect on agreed therapy goals can help keep therapeutic focus. As well us needing to understand the client's goals, to be helpful, the supervisor also needs to understand the supervisees goals for supervision. To model the importance of goals in therapy the supervisor may want start each supervision session by hearing the supervisee's goals for the supervision session.

> The supervisor might start by saying: so, we have about an hour for supervision today – what are your goals for the next hour? What do you want to get from it to have made it a useful hour?

In this example the supervisee expressed that they were feeling particularly stuck with a client and their goal was to get some ideas about how to proceed with the therapy. During the initial discussion about the case the supervisor heard that the client had a history of self-harm and had been referred to the service after a severe episode in which she had required hospitalization for treatment to some deep cuts. The supervisor heard that the client attended regularly but felt that she was not fully engaged in the therapy and was often quiet and noncommittal—the supervisor felt they were working increasingly hard to keep the session flowing and keep the client engaged.

SUPERVISOR: What have you been working on together?

SUPERVISEE: She is very risky and we have been working on a keep safe plan— to cut in a less dangerous way so she doesn't end up back in hospital.

SUPERVISOR: Is that what she wants?

SUPERVISEE: Yes—she frightened herself with the time she was admitted— she is very clear she doesn't want to end up back at A&E.

At this point in the supervision there was some further discussion around risk management—but the supervisor felt the therapist and the understandable anxiety in the system might drive the focus on risk. The supervisor wondered if the keep safe goals were truly shared by the client. The discussion returned to goals:

SUPERVISOR: You are very clear that a focus of the work should be on risk management and it seems quite right that it should and the client has been clear with you that they also want to stay safe and out of hospital—but what else do you think they want? If she were here in the room with us and we asked her what she wanted to change in her life, what she wanted to be better or different, what might she say?

SUPERVISEE: I think she would say that she wants a better relationship with her mother, she wants to go back to work.

SUPERVISOR: … and if you asked her to rank her goals—say which ones were the most important to her—where would keeping safe come in the list?

SUPERVISEE: I think she sees keeping safe to be a thing she *has* to do, the others are things she *wants* to do. …

SUPERVISOR: How much have you talked about the things she wants to do? Have a better relationship with her mum and get a job?

SUPERVISEE: The focus has been on keeping safe—so not much time has been spent on the other things. …

What has been uncovered here, through simply asking the supervisee to focus back on the client's goals, is that the supervisee has been focused on the risk management goals—these were clearly agreed goals and were undoubtedly the issue to focus on at the start of the intervention. As time moved on, however, the continued sole focus on this goal seems to have obscured the more important, higher order goals that the client had: relationship and job—perhaps leading to what the supervisee experienced as the partial engagement of the client. After further discussion, the supervisee decided to spend time in the next session exploring the client's higher order goals alongside the risk management goals. Returning to the goals of supervision set at the start of the session—the supervisee felt that the discussion had been helpful in reaching their supervision goal of feeling less stuck with this client.

Similar approaches can be used in consultation—where a practitioner might be invited to facilitate more of a psychological perspective on a family or individual that they do not see directly themselves. Often clinical consultations are sought when the system (those who work closely with the client) feel stuck. As with the previous example, an exploration of the goals of the system and how well these overlap with the goals of the person themselves can be a very simple and yet effective line of enquiry. These lines of enquiry can help the system see where its goals might obscure the goals of the client. For example in the world of looked-after children (LAC), often the system's primary goal is to reduce placement breakdown—this is usually in the best interest of the child and no doubt a good system goal to have. For the child, however, this might not be consciously high on their list of goals—they may see having freedom to see their friends as high on their list of goals. It is fine for these goals of the system and the child to be different—as long as both are held in mind. Part of the consultant's task in some stuck cases is to help the system explore these goals.

As with supervision, it can help the consultant model the goal-oriented practice by asking the individual or individual they are consulting to, to set goals for the consultation by asking: 'What will make this a helpful hour to spend together?' or 'If this turns out to be a helpful consultation—what do you hope to be different at the end of it?'. It is possible to use goal-based outcome tools at the beginning and the end of the consultation to track how useful the consultation has been in helping reach these goals. Simply inviting the system to explore the client's goals—and again asking them to rate how close to their goal the client might feel they are—can help the system move away from its own focus to understand the situation from others' perspectives—to mentalize—and therefore can help in moving to work more collaboratively with them.

Conclusion

Goal-oriented practice is a stance and not a therapy model. It draws on the evidence base as that is what is most likely to make therapy and therapeutic services effective and efficient. Its emphasis is on co-producing explicit goals for therapy that can then be revisited and tracked throughout an intervention. With some clients and with some modalities, goals might be helpfully referred to and monitored explicitly each session; with other clients and other interventions it could be weeks or months between explicit references back to goals. How often goals are explicitly referred to is less relevant than how much they are kept in mind by the therapist and the client—at each therapy session the implicit question should be asked: 'Why are we meeting again today, what are the goals, and how will what we do today help us work together to reach those goals?'.

Goal-oriented practice is simple to conceive but deceptively sophisticated and difficult to apply. We need to be realistic and pragmatic about the goals that are achievable in therapy and we certainly need to remain cognizant and conscious to the complexity and adversity in the real-world contexts in which many of our clients strive to reach their goals. Goal-oriented practice makes no claims at being *the* essential ingredient of therapy—but there is no doubt that it is one of the essential ingredients.

Points for reflection

♦ Thinking about your own practice—how much do you feel you adopt a goal-oriented practice approach in your own work?

♦ How can you ensure that you are co-producing goals that are genuinely shared and collaborative (and not just driven by your agenda or the agenda for the setting in which you work)? How can you test this out? Who can help?

♦ Look back at the transcripts in this chapter—what do you feel was good and what might you do or say differently if you were the therapist?

Acknowledgements

Thanks to Mick Cooper and Ann York for invaluable input into earlier drafts of this chapter and to Kate Martin and Jenna Jacob for developing these ideas with me over the years.

Further reading

Duncan, B. L., Miller, S. D., Wampold, B. E., & Hubble, M. A. (2010) (Eds.) *The Heart & Soul of Change: Delivering What Works in Therapy*. (2nd Edition). Washington, DC : APA.

Fonagy, P., Cottrell, D., Phillips, J., Bevington, D., Glaser, D., & Allison, E. (2014). *What works for whom?: a critical review of treatments for children and adolescents*. New York, NY: Guilford Publications.

References

Bateman, A. W., & Fonagy, P. (Eds.). (2012). *Handbook of mentalizing in mental health practice*. Arlington VA: American Psychiatric Association Publishing.

Bickman, L., Kelley, S. D., Breda, C., de Andrade, A. R., & Riemer, M. (2011). Effects of routine feedback to clinicians on mental health outcomes of youths: results of a randomized trial. *Psychiatric Services, 62*(12), 1423–9.

Bohart, A. C., & Tallman, K. (2010). Clients: The neglected common factor in psychotherapy. In Duncan, B. L. Miller, S. D., Wampold, B. E., Hubble, M. A. (Eds.), *The Heart & Soul of Change: Delivering What Works in Therapy* (2nd ed., pp. 83–112). Washington, DC: APA.

Bordin, E. S. (1979). The generalizability of the psychoanalytic concept of the working alliance. *Psychotherapy: Theory, Research & Practice, 16*(3), 252.

Chorpita., B, & Weisz., J. (2009). *MATCH-ADTC: Modular Approach to Therapy for Children with Anxiety, Depression, Trauma, or Conduct Problems*. Practice Wise: Florida.

Cohen, J. A., Berliner, L., & Mannarino, A. (2010). Trauma focused CBT for children with co-occurring trauma and behavior problems. *Child Abuse & Neglect, 34*(4), 215–24.

Cooper, M., & McLeod, J. (2011). Person-centered therapy: A pluralistic perspective. *Person-Centered & Experiential Psychotherapies, 10*(3), 210–23.

Department of Health (2009). *Reference guide to consent for examination or treatment*. (2nd Edition). London: Department of Health.

de Shazer, S. (1991). *Putting difference to work*. New York: Norton.

Division of Clinical Psychology. (2011). *Good practice guidelines on the use of psychological formulation*. Leicester: The British Psychological Society.

Edwards, A., & Elwyn, G. (2009). *Shared decision-making in health care: Achieving evidence-based patient choice*. Oxford University Press.

Holtforth, M. G., & Michalak, J. (2012). 25 Motivation in Psychotherapy. In Ryan R. M., (Ed.), *The Oxford Handbook of Human Motivation* (pp. 439–462). Oxford, UK: Oxford Handbook of Human Motivation.

Horvath, A. O., Del Re, A. C., Fluckinger, C., & Symonds, D. (2011). Alliance in individual psychotherapy. In J. C. Norcross (Ed.), *Psychotherapy Relationships that Work: Evidence-based responsiveness* (2nd ed., pp. 25–69). New York: Oxford University Press.

Lambert, M. J. (2005). Emerging methods for providing clinicians with timely feedback on treatment effectiveness: An introduction. *Journal of Clinical Psychology*, *61*(2), 141–4.

Law, D., & Bradley, J. (2013). *Goals and goal based outcomes (GBOs): Some useful information*. Version 3. CAMHS Press: London.

Milne, D. (2009). *Evidence-based clinical supervision*. Chichester: BPS Blackwell.

NHS Digital (2016). *Psychological Therapies: Annual report on the use of IAPT services 2015-16*. Health and Social Care Information Centre.

Orlinsky, D. E.; Rønnestad, M. H.; Willutzki, U. (2004*).* Fifty years of psychotherapy process-outcomes research: Continuity and change. In M. J. Lambert, (Ed.). *Bergin and Garfield's Handbook of Psychotherapy and Behavior Change* (pp. 307–93). New York: Wiley.

Roth, A., & Fonagy, P. (2013). *What works for whom?: a critical review of psychotherapy research*. New York, NY: Guilford Publications.

Tryon, G. S., & Winograd, G. (2011). Goal consensus and collaboration. *Psychotherapy*, *48*(1), 50–7.

Weisz, J. R., Chorpita, B. F., Frye, A., Ng, M. Y., Lau, N., Bearman, S. K., Ugueto, A.M., Langer, D.A., & Hoagwood, K. E.; Research Network on Youth Mental Health. (2011). Youth Top Problems: using idiographic, consumer-guided assessment to identify treatment needs and to track change during psychotherapy. *Journal of Consulting and Clinical Psychology*, *79*(3), 369.

Wolpert, M. (2016). Failure is an option. *The Lancet Psychiatry*, *3*(6), 510–12.

Wolpert, M., Ford, T., Trustam, E., Law, D., Deighton, J., Flannery, H., & Fugard, R. J. (2012). Patient-reported outcomes in child and adolescent mental health services (CAMHS): Use of idiographic and standardized measures. *Journal of Mental Health*, *21*(2), 165–73.

Wolpert, M., Jacob, J., Napoleone, E., Whale, A., Calderon, J., & Edbrooke-Childs, J. (2016). *Child and Parent-reported Outcomes and Experience from Child and Young People's Mental Health Services 2011-2015* CAMHS Press: London.

York, A., & Kingsbury, S. (2013). *The Choice and Partnership Approach: A service transformation model*. Surrey: CAPA Systems Limited.

Chapter 9

Goal-oriented practice across therapies

Nick Grey, Suzanne Byrne,
Tracey Taylor, Avi Shmueli, Cathy Troupp,
Peter Stratton, Aaron Sefi, Roslyn Law,
and Mick Cooper

The goal of this chapter is to consider goal-oriented practices from the perspective of the principal therapeutic orientations, and the distinctive ways in which goal-oriented practices may be applied in these approaches. Specifically, this chapter focuses on:

- cognitive behaviour therapy;
- psychoanalytic psychotherapy and psychoanalysis;
- psychoanalytic child psychotherapy;
- systemic family therapy;
- online therapy;
- interpersonal psychotherapy;
- humanistic and existential therapies.

Cognitive behaviour therapy

Nick Grey, Suzanne Byrne, Tracey Taylor

Cognitive behavioural therapies are a family of therapies that share many common conceptual underpinnings, while often differing in emphases and techniques used. Over time these therapies have evolved from early behavioural therapies, to the integration of a more cognitive emphasis, and more recently the development of contextual behavioural therapies, sometimes referred to as 'third wave'. There is substantial evidence that CBT is an effective treatment for a wide range of presenting problems (Westbrook, Kennerley, & Kirk, 2011).

A foundation of CBT is that an individual's thoughts, emotions, behaviour, and bodily reactions are integrally linked, set within an environment or context, including interpersonal context (Beck, 2011). Altering any one part of the system allows there to be changes in other aspects. Thoughts are taken to mean not only the actual explicit thoughts that go through someone's mind, but also include terms such as beliefs and appraisals, which may be implicit and reflect underlying meanings for the person. In addition, meanings may be associated with and reflected by images that people experience.

A key tenet of CBT is that of 'collaborative empiricism'. This reflects the therapeutic relationship ideally being that of partners working together, and close attention should be paid to the impact of whatever work the therapy entails, on various levels, such as symptoms, functioning, and quality of life. CBT is typically short term, 10-12 sessions, although longer CBT treatment is not uncommon in more complicated cases, and even shorter interventions based on CBT principles are increasingly widespread in stepped care health services (Richards & McDonald, 1990).

Goals in CBT

CBT therapists focus on developing a shared understanding of a person's current difficulties with a formulation/conceptualization. The client and therapist then consider goals alongside this—turning problems into goals. The aim is to have clear mutually agreed goals that therapy will focus on helping client to work toward. The advantages of this are that: it helps to foster a sense of hope and reduce helplessness; it helps give therapy a focus and direction to be working towards; it helps to consider what is achievable in the time available; it helps to develop a sense of collaboration.

Setting goals in CBT

Goals will be discussed in CBT from the first meeting with a client and these are agreed at different time points depending on the individual. For example, when working with people with OCD, discussion of alternative less-threatening explanations for their experiences occurs early in therapy. It is only once the client is able to even consider such an alternative perspective to their problem that it is possible for them to see what goals for therapy may include (Challacombe, Bream, & Salkovskis, 2011).

Clients are encouraged to have goals that are positively stated and focused on observable behavioural change, that is 'what will you be doing that will be different?'. Like many other therapy modalities, the 'SMART' acronym is used as the basis for goal setting (specific, measurable, achievable, realistic, time-limited;

see also Chapter 7, this volume). Some examples of questions to help elicit goals are outlined below:

◆ What would you be able to do if the problem improved?
◆ What would you like to do in the future that you cannot do now because of the problem?
◆ What would you like to be doing by the end of therapy?
◆ How would you know when the problem has been resolved or improved?
◆ How will you know you are making progress?

Goals are written down with both client and therapist having a record of these to refer back to. Clients are asked to rate their current success on a rating scale, that is 'Where would you rate yourself now on a scale of 0-10?'.

Clients are encouraged to break goals down into composite steps, focusing on short-term goals initially and also considering medium- and longer-term goals.

Short-term goals are usually main priorities to start working on, or areas in which a client wishes to see immediate change, or may be less difficult goals, things that the client feels fairly confident they could achieve if they put their mind to them. These should be achievable within the first few weeks of therapy and can include attending therapy appointments.

Medium-term goals may be slightly more difficult to achieve, may require more work, but are things that the client would like to see changing during therapy, or the follow-up period, for example 'Every week taking my baby to playgroup, playing with the other children and enjoying my time there'.

Long-term goals are often the things that the client might have stopped thinking about because of their problems. Individuals are encouraged to see that these are their hopes and dreams for the future and often these have been abandoned, neglected, or seen as impossible. No matter how dejected a client might feel about the problem, it is important to help them to think of how they would like to be, what they would like to be doing, what life would look like if they didn't have this problem, for example 'To pursue a career in child care'.

Using goals in CBTs

Goals in CBT are not static and are revised and refined as therapy progresses. Regular reviews take place with the client re-rating their degree of success in achieving their goal.

CBT therapies have specific aims, which vary depending on the setting and type of CBT being offered. Therapists will consider treatment goals in the context of their client's current level of distress and functioning during therapy. Potential priorities for therapy will be discussed with clients, for example to reduce suicidal risk in depression. In dialectical behaviour therapy there are hierarchies of goals set by the framework of the treatment, in which addressing self-harm is always the primary goal. In acceptance and commitment therapy there is explicit work on identifying a person's values, and 'goals' are higher level such as 'acceptance' or 'willingness', which are deliberately less SMART than in other forms of CBT. This is also true to some extent of other therapies such as mindfulness based cognitive therapy (see Westbrook *et al.*, 2011).

In group CBT there will be group goals set alongside individual goals. Goal-setting with children and adolescents will often more explicitly include discussions with parents, and others in the young person's system such as teachers.

Therapist goals in CBT

Goals are also integral to CBT training, for therapist and supervisor development. Goal-setting is a key competency for CBT therapists and supervisors to master. Additionally, therapists and supervisors in training and when qualified are encouraged to develop their own learning goals along the principles outlined above, for example 'to be able to use socratic questioning with my clients, to be able to develop my case formulation skills in depression' (Roth & Pilling, 2007).

Summary

Goals are an integral part of CBT. They provide the direction for a therapy that is usually short term and problem focused. Goals are typically set collaboratively by the person (or persons) and the therapist. Goals are set for sessions using agendas, for the duration of the treatment, and for beyond treatment in to the future. Goals are reviewed and revised as necessary during treatment. Therapists and supervisors are also encouraged to use goals for their own development.

References

Beck, J. S. (2011). *Cognitive Therapy: Basics and Beyond.* 2nd Edition. New York: Guilford Press.

Challacombe, F., Bream, V., & Salkovskis, P. (2011). *Break Free from OCD.* London: Vermillion.

Westbrook, D., Kennerley, H., & Kirk, J. (2011). *An Introduction to Cognitive Behaviour Therapy: Skills and Applications*, 2nd Ed. London: Sage Publications.

Psychoanalytic Psychotherapy and Psychoanalysis

Avi Shmueli

It was probably Sigmund Freud's initial training as a physician, coupled with his capacity for close observation as illustrated by his drawings of neurones, that led him to develop psychoanalysis as a theory of mental functioning using the concepts of form and function. Based on his theory of the instincts, the Topographical Model of the mind (which defined the conscious, preconscious, and unconscious systems, Freud, 1900), and the Structural Model (which defined the agencies of the Id, Ego, and Superego, Freud, 1923), psychoanalytic theory has further developed into a number of different schools of thought. The Contemporary Freudian, Independent, and Kleinian schools nevertheless retain fundamental psychoanalytic assumptions all of which can be traced back to Freud.

The mind from a psychoanalytic view is an entity that is first and foremost developing and developmental so that a continuity exists between what has occurred previously and the present. Consequently, the complexity and multiplicity of processes in the unconscious system are responsible for much of the content of conscious experience. Conscious experience itself, including symptomatology, is overdetermined, that is has multiple meanings as many aspects of subjective experience are simultaneously expressed. Psychic conflict is therefore not only inevitable but ubiquitous, the extent, intensity, and expression of which is influenced by adverse events in childhood. The unresolved aspects of the past are considered to be unconsciously and compulsively repeated in the present in an attempt at resolution (Freud, 1920). The mind therefore also functions to maximize psychic safety and manage extremes of both pleasure and what is termed as 'unpleasure'. The role of defence mechanisms is crucial and these are respected clinically rather than automatically assumed to be deleterious to functioning. The fundamental relational nature of both intra-psychic and inter-psychic experience implies that the relationship between patient and therapist be the most important forum for therapeutic change, that is working in what is termed the Transference.

The structure and functioning of the mind led Freud to be overly concise regarding goals for treatment, both colloquially, in saying the individual should aim 'to be able to love and to work' (Freud, 1950), and also in terms of theory by stating that the aim of treatment would be to make the unconscious conscious and that 'where id there shall ego be' (Freud, 1933). This latter statement, with its implicit emphasis on increasingly developed mastery and refined expression of unconscious wishes, was expanded by Knight (1941) and Ross (1963) into terms more recognizable to current clinicians. In the course of psychotherapy, three different realms of development may be evidenced to differing extents depending on the setting of the treatment itself. First, the disappearance of the presenting symptoms as these are essentially an acceptable expression of what had up to now been experienced as an unacceptable underlying wish and/or conflict. Second, an improvement in aspects of mental functioning such as the capacity to tolerate different affects and internal conflicts without having to translate these into potentially self-damaging behaviours. This would require the development of greater insight and would also lead to a greater acceptance of oneself and appreciation of strengths as well as weaknesses. Third, and concomitantly, there would be an improved adjustment to external reality in terms of the quality of relationships, the capacity to work and to be creative. Bernardi (2001) most clearly cites Bleger's (1973) distinction between curative goals which focus on the alleviation of subjective suffering, and goals which aim at the 'enrichment of a more complete development'.

It becomes clear that psychoanalysis has universal goals for all patients, these being related to aspects of unconscious functioning and underlying psychic structure. Simultaneously, therapist-set, manifest goals for psychoanalytically based therapies are, however, problematic. The psychoanalytic model explicitly gives precedence to unconscious functioning and essentially views conscious report and behaviour as representative of such unconscious functioning. The emphasis on the transference relationship and the stance required by the therapist of goalessness (Wallerstein, 1965), or having free-floating attention (Sandler, 1976), or being 'without memory or desire' (Bion, 1970), are consistent with the therapist being available to be directed by the patient's unconscious functioning, as represented by their consciously spoken free associations, to the unconscious meaning of the patient's functioning. Goal-setting by the therapist for a patient, which can only be consciously done, would powerfully interfere with the therapist's central task.

However, just as the patient is at liberty to say whatever comes to mind, so the patient is free to express their own hopes fears and goals for their own therapy. It is true that many individuals seek psychoanalytic psychotherapy and psychoanalysis simply because they wish to 'feel better' or because they need 'help'. However, others also seek help with specific goals; better relationships, specific relationships, achieving or minimizing aspects of sexuality and sexual practice, unrealized ambitions, or the wish for relief from intense feelings such as depression, dread, emptiness, anxiety, and so forth. Patient-led goals are readily accepted as by definition they are considered to be important and disguised representations of unconscious fixations and or conflicts. Indeed, in some cases goals and the patient's vicissitudes in achieving them may serve as a good barometer of change and development.

The Tavistock Adult Depression Study (Fonagy *et al.*, 2015) is one of the best examples of the achievement of goals in the absence of them being explicitly and formally set by the therapist. In a randomized controlled trial, adults with chronic and treatment-resistant depression received 18 months of once-weekly psycho-analytic psychotherapy compared with a control group receiving treatment rec-ommended in the NICE guidelines. At a two-year follow-up, 44% of the therapy sample no longer met the criteria for major depression compared with 10% of the control sample. Additionally, those in the treatment sample evidenced sig-nificant benefits to their quality of life and social and personal functioning. The Fonagy *et al.* (2015) study may therefore be more of an example of Wallerstein's (1965) distinction between outcome goals, phrased in terms of symptomatology and not usually set in psychoanalytic psychotherapy, as opposed to other thera-pies and process goals which are descriptions of psychic functioning embedded in a theory of change.

References

Bernardi, R. (2001) Psychoanalytic Goals: new and Old Paradoxes. *Psychoanalytic Quarterly, 70,* 67–98.

Bleger, J. (1973). Criterios de curación y objetivos del psicoanálisis. *Revista de Psicoanálisis, 30(2),* 317–50.

Bion, W.R. *Attention and Interpretation: A Scientific Approach to Insight in Psycho-Analysis and Groups.* London: Tavistock. 1970.

Fonagy, P., Rost, F. Carlyle, J. McPherson, S., Thomas, R., Fearon, P., Goldberg, D, Taylor, D. (2015). Pragmatic randomized controlled trial of long-term psychoanalytic psychotherapy for treatment-resistant depression: the Tavistock Adult Depression Study (TADS). *World Psychiatry, 14,* 312–21.

Fonagy, P., Steele, M., Steele, H., Leigh, T., Kennedy, R., Mattoon, G., Target, M. (1995). Attachment, the reflective self, and borderline states; the predictive specificity of the adult attachment interview and pathological emotional development. In S. Goldberg *et al.* (Ed.), *Attachment Theory: Social, Developmental and Clinical Perspectives* (pp. 233–76). New York: Academic Press.

Freud, S. (1900) The Interpretation of Dreams. *S.E.,* 4-5.

Freud, S. (1920) Beyond the Pleasure Principle. *S.E.,* 18.

Freud, S. (1923) The Ego and the Id. *S.E.,* 19.

Freud, S. (1933). New introductory lectures on psycho-analysis. *S.E.,* 22, p. 80.

Freud, S. (1950) quoted by E. H. Erikson: Growth and crises of the healthy personality In *Problems of Infancy and Childhood* New York: Josiah Macy, Jr. Foundation, 1950, p. 141.

Knight, R. P. (1941-1942). Evaluation of the results of psychoanalytic therapy. *Amer. J. Psychiatry,* **98,** 434–46.

Ross, N. (1963) Aims and goals of psychoanalytic therapy: clinical and metapsychological descriptions. Presented at the panel on the Theory of Psychoanalytic Therapy, Midwinter Meeting, American Psychoanalytic Association, 7 December 1963.

Sandler, J. (1976) Countertransference and Role-Responsiveness. *International Review of Psycho-Analysis, 3,* 33–47.

Wallerstein, R. S. (1965). The Goals of Psychoanalysis—A survey of Analytic Viewpoints. *Journal of the American Psychoanalytic Association, 13,* 748–70.

Psychoanalytic child psychotherapy

Cathy Troupp

Psychoanalytic child psychotherapy (from here referred to as just child psychotherapy) is a hybrid, with its roots in adult psychoanalysis and its practice embedded in modern child and adolescent mental health; the result is an endemic tension between theory and practice. At best, this tension results in flexible, imaginative, and child-centred therapies that focus on bringing the voice of the child to the complex networks around vulnerable children, such as looked-after children, or children with environmental and developmental histories that have led to difficulties with self-expression and individuation.

Child psychotherapists have largely embraced goal-setting in the past decade. Its value lies particularly in bringing focus and a shared task to an open, exploratory therapy. Its role in tracking whether young people are achieving hoped-for change is also crucial in child psychotherapy as in all therapies. As there has been no guidance on best practice for implementing goal-setting in clinical practice, child psychotherapists are likely to be varying in the way they set goals.

There are a couple of potential theoretical and technical obstacles to goal-setting in child psychotherapy. Equally, there are some particular strengths and advantages that child psychotherapy can bring to goal-based practice.

First, psychoanalytic therapy, including child psychotherapy, traditionally prioritizes the 'inner world' and, furthermore, the 'unconscious'. Clearly, it is not possible to set goals relating to the unconscious as it is, by its own terms, inaccessible to conscious awareness.

However, a therapist who closely tracks the young person's narrative, uses clarifying questions, and tentative probes aimed at prompting new thoughts about self and other, can lead to what was previously 'unconscious'. This way, goals can relate to the 'inner world' of a young person, their very personal experiences, and their wishes for change.

Further, child psychotherapists focus on the 'inner world' as well as on the 'outer world' and naturally recognize the interplay between the two and the way in which what was unconscious or semi-conscious can be brought to conscious awareness through therapeutic conversation. So there are many opportunities and arenas for goal-setting.

Like all therapies, child psychotherapy aims to facilitate change. Traditionally, the model of how change happens has been broad brush, with the emphasis being on the therapeutic relationship as the vehicle of change. In this sense, psychodynamic practice prioritizes the therapeutic alliance that is at the heart of goal-setting in psychotherapy. The therapist working with 'the unconscious' will likely be able to help the young person to elucidate and articulate their wish for change even when these wishes may be mere seedlings underground at the start of therapy, allowing for the elucidation of deeply, personally, meaningful goals.

Second, psychoanalytic psychotherapy has traditionally eschewed directive discussion and engagement with the 'outer world'. Psychoanalytic therapists prefer to refrain from giving advice (Blagys & Hilsenroth, 2000; Schneider *et al.*, 2009). Unlike cognitive and behavioural therapies, psychodynamic therapy avoids homework tasks or other directive involvement with the young person's relationships and environment. This may make the formulation of goals more difficult in the immediate term, but on the other hand, the therapist's reticence to take on advice giving can open the space for the young person to take more responsibility for formulating their own goals, particularly when scaffolded by their therapist. This can happen, for example, by means of iterative conversation in the early stages of therapy or assessment for therapy, around a particular topic, until the therapist feels confident to suggest that this issue may be suitable for goal-setting.

The 'model' of goal-setting where the goals are collaboratively worked up between therapist and young person in the course of the first few sessions (Law, 2011) fits the child psychotherapy model well, insofar as the therapist follows the young person's lead in keeping with the original idea of 'free association', and unlike cognitive and behavioural therapies, prefers to avoid structuring the session (Schneider *et al.*, 2009).

I have written about my own preference for working up 'dual goals' (Troupp, 2013, 2014). By this I mean that a goal about hoped-for changes in the young person's inner world, changes in their feelings or emotions, or ways of relating to others, can then be given a second part by asking the question, 'How would you know when your goal had been achieved?'. Dual goals create links between the inner world of emotion and thought, to the outer world of behavioural change. This way, goals can remain congruent with the young person's emotional, developmental concerns at a deep level, while also providing practical and behavioural foci, as illustrated by the following case example.

Freya, a young woman of 16, started psychotherapy in the wake of her physical recovery from an eating disorder, having expressed a wish to learn to become more emotionally aware. Her mother had died the previous year after several years of suffering from cancer and enduring debilitating chemotherapy. Freya lived with her widowed father, who had just begun a new relationship. She was beginning to formulate a theory that her own feelings had had to go 'on ice' during the whole of this period.

After a couple of exploratory sessions with her therapist, her 'dual goals' looked like this:

Freya's goals		Rating at Time 1	Rating at Time 2 (after six months of therapy)
Part 1: 'inner world' change	Part 2: behavioural change		
1. Feel less guilty about leaving Dad	Go out with my friends more	3	[8]
2. Continue recovery from eating disorder	Relax my rules around eating - range and times	5	[7]
3. Understand why I have panic attacks	Be able to use strategies to help myself when I feel panicky	3	[9]

It can be seen that the goals were based on Freya's level of self-awareness at the point at which therapy began. The goals were drawn from the struggles of which she was conscious. There was at this time no 'goal' relating to grieving for her mother. A therapist might reasonably think that grieving might be an essential process, and indeed through the course of therapy Freya talked about many things related to her mother's illness and death, but it was an organic process and at this time perhaps not amenable to goal-setting.

After six months, when the goals were reviewed for the second time, in accordance with the practice of the CAMH service, Freya rated them at 8, 7, and 9, respectively.

Regarding Goal 1, Freya was going out more with friends and consciously felt less guilty about her father.

Regarding Goal 2, Freya's eating disorder was more under her control but not totally—the psychological component of an eating disorder may remain part of a young person's thinking many years after physical recovery.

Regarding Goal 3, things had improved significantly, in that Freya had not suffered panic attacks for several months. It seemed likely that some work done with her therapist relating to the panic attacks to the loss of her mother had helped make sense of the symptom; equally, her livelier social circle meant that she was less likely to be out on her own—an example of a positive 'eco-cycle' of change.

At the review, Freya noted that the goals set no longer captured her primary preoccupations, as the conversations in therapy, and her own process, had brought her to a place where she was beginning to want to move on from living in the shadow of the loss of her mother. She expressed this in many ways, both contradictory and linear, and introduced a new goal which was not to feel guilty about 'moving on'. The behavioural part of this goal she set as doing new things—things that her mother would not now see.

Goal-setting in therapy has been welcomed and embraced by many psychoanalytic and psychodynamic practitioners as a way of bringing focus and clarity to interventions, both for the therapist and the young person (Emanuel *et al.*, 2013). A therapist who approaches the young person's concerns with respectful curiosity, maintains uncertainty, listens carefully to current concerns, and explores wished for changes at both the manifest and below-the-surface levels, should have little difficulty in helping a young person to find meaningful personal goals for change.

References

Blagys, M.D., & Hilsenroth, M.J. (2000). Distinctive Features of Short-Term Psychodynamic-Interpersonal Psychotherapy: A Review of the Comparative Psychotherapy Process Literature. *Clinical Psychology: Science and Practice, 7(2)*, 167–88.

Emanuel, R., Catty, J., Anscombe, E., Cantle, A., & Muller, H. (2013). 'Implementing an aim-based outcome measure in a psychoanalytic child psychotherapy service: insights, experiences and evidence'. *Clinical Child Psychology & Psychiatry, 19(2)*, 169–83.

Law, D. (2011). *Goals and Goal Based Outcomes (GBOs) version 2.0—some useful information*. CAMHS Press: London

Schneider, C., Pruetzel-Thomas, A., & Midgley, N. (2009). Discovering New Ways of Seeing and Speaking about Psychotherapy Process: the Child Psychotherapy Q-Set. In eds. Midgley, N., Anderson, J., Grainger, E., Nesic-Vuckovic, T. and Urwin, C. *Child Psychotherapy and Research: New Approaches, Emerging Findings*. Routledge, Hove, East Sussex.

Troupp, C. (2013). 'What do you want to get from coming here?' Distinguishing patient-generated outcome measures in CAMHS from a bespoke sandwich. *Child and Family Clinical Psychology Review, 1(1)*, 19–28.

Troupp, C. (2014). Clinical commentary. *Journal of Child Psychotherapy, 40*, 1,

Systemic family therapy

Peter Stratton

The therapeutic model

Systemic family therapists (SFT) may work with individuals, couples, families, and other constellations of close relationships, but are always focused on the role of close relationships in the presenting problem. The SFT stance sees quality of functioning of relationships as fundamental to the psychological health of the individual, and therefore concentrates on working with the patient in the context of those relationships. In many cases this is best achieved by having the partner or the family actively participating in the therapy. Most of the concepts discussed in this section are elaborated by Carr (2012) and in the overview of SFT and its current outcome evidence by Stratton (2016).

Conceptualizing goals in a systemic frame

Because SFT is more focused on establishing conditions for a better future, rather than finding explanations in the past for current problems, it is in many ways automatically focussing on goals. However, the concept of initial goal-setting does not resonate well with the kind of non-prescriptive approaches of current SFT. SFT places a high value on side-stepping the therapist's norms and assumptions, and indeed the assumptions of family members, so early fixing on goals for the therapy is inappropriate. It is our experience that an initial specification of the problem by a referrer or a family member, will change radically as the work of building a systemic understanding develops throughout therapy.

Models of family therapy (FT) vary in how specifically they define their goals. From experiential FT where the main therapeutic goal is the growth of each family member as a whole person rather than the resolution of specific problems, through the common approach where the resolution of symptoms is the main goal, to those that focus on concrete behaviours, for example Not that 'we get on better', but 'we go out together once a week'.

One example of a way to achieve a concrete description of a goal is the 'miracle question' from solution-focused therapy: 'If you woke up tomorrow and the problem had gone, what would each member of the family notice as being different?' (de Shazer, 1988). Other therapies, of the form labelled 'strategic', look for agreement on the smallest change that will make a difference:

> The following goal-setting questions involve asking clients about the minimum degree of change that would need to occur for them to believe that they had begun the journey down the road to problem resolution:
> - What is the first thing I would notice if I walked into your house if things were just beginning to change for the better?
> - What is the smallest thing that would have to change for you to know you were moving in the right direction to solve this difficult problem?
>
> (Carr, 2012, p. 245)

Setting goals

In an early paper in this area, Carr (1993) showed how established findings from studies of goal-setting in occupational and industrial contexts could be applied in SFT. He concluded on the importance of participation in goal-setting, seeing therapy as a cooperative and open venture rather than a competitive and deceptive enterprise.

One example of a collaborative approach is to invite the family to together describe how they hope the family would be in the future: 'Imagine five years have passed, you are (give each their age then)—how would you hope the family would look?'. Out of this discussion, the family will consider stages to move them towards such a future, ending with an agreement about what they need to be able to do now. These discussions not only generate the immediate goals, but also give the therapist a guide to more fundamental changes that the family might make in how it operates. An early recognition in the field was the value of going beyond the changes that could be achieved within the system's current rules (first order change) and working with the family system to change its rules (second order change), which can be expected to have more radical and long-lasting effects, (see Carr, 2012, p. 98). The current orientation to strengths and solutions leads to opening up agreements about goals. Some therapists will primarily focus on drawing out a recognition of the potential of the family, and how they can keep the positives as a more powerful aspect of their identity and expectations. Others will proceed to making the goals explicit, so defining the immediate objectives of the therapy.

While many in SFT treat the goals of therapy as a product of the therapeutic process, the context of the work will often impose goals. For example, if a juvenile is referred by the courts for drug offences, an obvious goal will be reduced substance abuse, but in family work the most important goal may emerge when a programme has been completed. Dakof *et al.* (2015) report that it was the reduction in criminal behaviour, sustained for 24 months, that was ultimately seen as most valuable.

Use of goals through therapy

People who attend for SFT often bring a symptomatic behaviour of one person in the relationship as their goal for therapy. As the therapy proceeds, the focus on how the relationships have operated and how changes in the ways that relationships are implemented could have positive consequences for everyone, will hopefully broaden the perception of goals in the way labelled above as 'second order change'.

In common with other psychotherapies, SFT recognizes that the quality of the therapeutic alliance underpins the achievement of more specific goals, and the building of the alliance has particular significance, and particular challenges, when working with a family (Karam, Sprenkle, & Davis, 2015). But the alliance can also be an outcome of successful work towards defining more functional goals. In their qualitative metasynthesis of 49 articles centred on clients' experiences of their conjoint couple and family therapy, Chenail *et al.* (2012) found that the collaborative process with all participants of agreeing on goals is itself a valuable process to meet the objectives of SFT "especially when this process was perceived as being collaborative and fitting with clients' understandings of their problems and core issues" (p. 252).

Conclusion

Setting goals at the start of therapy, as required by managed care, sits uneasily with the systemic view of goals emerging as part of the therapeutic process. We can identify two alternative responses. Research into the outcomes of SFT has primarily been in terms of specified conditions which could be seen as defining the goals of therapy. Stratton (2016) identified a total of 72 specified problems for which recent research had demonstrated that family therapy had been effective. It is clear that specific goals defined by the urgent concerns which bring people to therapy are important in the field, as shown by Carr's (2012) *Handbook* having 174 references to goals, indicating their use at every stage of the many approaches he describes. But the pattern in published research is perhaps driven by the dominant outcome paradigm. Within everyday practice, most clinics will see a great variety of families with a mixture of problems, often ill-defined. Rather than the proliferation of outcome measures identified by Stratton *et al.* (2015), an alternative has been to specify the goal of therapy in much broader terms by measuring improvement in the quality of close relationships. When a group of family therapists set out to create an outcome measure that would be applicable in all family therapies, they identified the functionality of the couple and family relationships as the most general goal. The measure they produced is the SCORE Index of Family Functioning and Change, which has consistently demonstrated positive outcomes of family therapy (Carr & Stratton, 2017; Stratton *et al.*, 2014).

So a general formulation of the goal of SFT could be that it works with families to adjust the operation of their relationships in ways that will equip them to more readily achieve their goals now and in the future.

References

Carr, A. (1993). Systemic consultation and goal setting. *Human Systems: The Journal of Systemic Consultation & Management, 4*, 49–59.

Carr, A. (2012). *Family Therapy: Concepts, Process and Practice* (3rd edn). Chichester: Wiley.

Carr, A., & Stratton, P. (2017). The Score Family Assessment Questionnaire: A Decade of Progress. *Fam. Proc., 56*, 285–301. doi:10.1111/famp.12280

Chenail, R.J., St. George, S., Wulff, D., Duffy, M., Wilson Scott, K., & Tomm, K. (2012). Clients' relational conceptions of conjoint couple and family therapy quality: A grounded formal theory. *Journal of Marital and Family Therapy, 38(1)*, 241–64.

Dakof, G.A., Henderson, C.E., Rowe, C.L., Boustani, M., Greenbaum, P.E., Wang, W., Hawes, S., Linares, C., & Liddle, H.A. (2015). A randomized clinical trial of family therapy in juvenile drug court. *Journal of Family Psychology, 29(2)*, 232–41.

Karam, E. A., Sprenkle, D. H., & Davis, S. D. (2015). Targeting threats to the therapeutic alliance: A primer for marriage and family therapy training. *Journal of Marital and Family Therapy, 41*, 389–400. doi: 10.1111/jmft.12097

de Shazer, S. (1988). *Clues: Investigating Solutions in Brief Therapy*. New York: Norton.

Stratton, P. (2016). *The Evidence Base of Family Therapy and Systemic Practice*. Association for Family Therapy, UK. Download at http://www.aft.org.uk/about/view/Research.html

Stratton, P., Silver, E. Nascimento, N. McDonnell L. Powell, G., & Nowotny, E. (2015). Couples and Family Therapy in the Previous Decade—What does the evidence tell us? *Contemporary Family Therapy, 27*, 1–12. doi: 10.1007/s10591-014-9314-6

Stratton, P., Lask, J., Bland, J., Nowotny, E., Evans, C., Singh, R., Janes, E., & Peppiatt, A. (2014). Validation of the SCORE-15 Index of Family Functioning and Change in detecting therapeutic improvement early in therapy. *Journal of Family Therapy, 36*, 3–19. doi: 10.1111/1467-6427.12022

Online therapy

Aaron Sefi

Online therapy has developed significantly in recent years, primarily through synchronous and asynchronous mail messaging, as well as video-conferencing. As part of a broader use of technology in therapy, it increasingly uses self-directed and self-help methods, such as through 'e-learning' packages and digital applications. These can often be administered alongside the therapist sessions and contact. Online therapy can be practiced privately, and increasingly through health funding, often in organizational contexts (Goss *et al.*, 2016).

The most critical feature of online therapy that can impact on goal-setting is probably the online disinhibition effect (Suler, 2004). On the one hand, this can make a client more honest about their goals, with the flip side being, where disinhibition is less benign, it can lead to fantastical or unrealistic goal-setting. Another feature is the accessibility and immediacy of online therapy, which can lead to different emphasis on types and categories of goals being identified online in contrast to face-to-face goals (Hanley *et al.*, 2016). The autonomous nature of the modality can also have an impact, where the power dynamic and how a bond develops through online contact can lead to a different kind of power dynamics in goal-setting and assessing. Finally the technology itself has its own impact, allowing goal-setting and progress checking to take place outside of the live contact. It can also be embedded into self-directed activity, such as through an application.

To illustrate these features, we can explore the case example of Sonya, a female in her early twenties. She was referred by her general practitioner to receive online therapy through an organization providing web-based and digital application-based therapy. She was suffering low-level post-natal depression and anxiety, and the accessibility and immediacy of the online modality appealed to her.

As part of a comprehensive assessment, and in developing rapport, Sonya and her therapist defined her life goals and therapy goals as:

1. to explore difficult feelings towards baby (therapy goal);
2. to communicate needs better to partner (life goal);
3. to develop confidence to reach out to other mums locally (life and therapy goal);

These goals were recorded and charted using CoGS (or Counselling Goals System—a specific goal-based outcome measure designed for online use, see Appendix 6.1, Chapter 6, this volume). Sonya received six live 'chat' sessions, interspersed with mail messaging and the self-directed use of an application over a period of three months. The measure indicated that, by end of therapy, she partly achieved Goal 2 (a 5-point movement out of 10), completely achieved Goal 3, but showed little movement towards Goal 1.

Initially, Sonya was very open and explicit about her difficult feelings, demonstrating the effects of online disinhibition. She sent numerous messages (some late at night) expressing some difficult feelings about her baby. However, during the live sessions, she seemed avoidant of the subject, and it was hard to bring attention back to it, without challenging the delicate bond that had been established. Here we can see how the asynchronous element of online therapy has a disinhibiting effect on goal-setting. The goal of exploring difficult feelings towards her baby was starting to be achieved in her messages, but then retracted during live sessions, reflecting Sonya's need to stay in control and her apparent lack of readiness to explore the issue in a more direct way.

Sonya preferred being task-oriented, and embraced the self-directed learning with gusto, regularly reporting positive benefits that related to communicating with her partner. In this, the power balance bore fruit. With Sonya feeling more in control she felt able to take the more 'manageable chunks' of talking to her partner, and reaching out to other mums locally.

The sense of autonomy offered by online therapy created an opportunity for Sonya to move quickly towards the goals she was prepared to achieve, and to avoid those she was not yet ready to face. This power dynamic also had an impact on the therapist's perception of the bond, as Sonya was able to control the depth of sessions, and consequently the goals she felt ready to work on.

At the end of their sessions, Sonya reported feeling a lot more in control of her life. But she still seemed reticent to explore where her difficult feelings and darker fantasies had come from, or where they had gone. This reflects how online therapy can increase the opportunity for expression of fantasy. If the bond is sufficient, a skilful online therapist can use creativity of fantasy to broaden the range of goal-setting. The challenge for the therapist is to ensure the goal-setting remains grounded in reality. In some cases fantasy can also lead to exaggeration around goal-setting that requires a similar reality check from the therapist.

Overall in this example, we can see how goal-setting and achievement can manifest in subtle, yet distinct ways in online therapy. The nature of online work can vary across clients, and through employing differing tasks and methods. However, the key unique elements of this medium are likely to impact in some form.

References

Goss, S., Anthony, K., Sykes Stretch, L., Merz Nagal, D. (2016) *Technology in Mental Health: Applications in Practice, Supervision and Therapy* 2nd Ed; Charles C Thomas: Illinois.

Hanley, T., Ersahin, Z., Sefi, A. & Hebron, J. (2016), Comparing Online and Face-to-Face Student Counselling: What Therapeutic Goals Are Identified and What Are the Implications for Educational Providers? *Journal of Psychologists and Counsellors in Schools.* DOI: 10.1017/jgc.2016.20

Suler, J. (2004). The online disinhibition effect. *Cyberpsychology & Behavior: The Impact of the Internet, Multimedia and Virtual Reality on Behavior and Society,* 7, 321–6. http://doi.org/10.1089/1094931041291295

Interpersonal psychotherapy

Roslyn Law

What is interpersonal psychotherapy?

Interpersonal psychotherapy (IPT, Markowitz & Weissman *et al.*, 2012) is a time-limited, structured treatment for depression, originally developed for use with adults and subsequently adapted for use across the life span (Mufson, Pollack, & Dorta, 2004; Dietz *et al.*, 2015). IPT's central idea is that problems in interpersonal relationships foster and maintain depressive symptoms in a bidirectional interaction. IPT provides scaffolding for change through enhancing social support and social learning, interpersonal problem solving and communication skills training. These changes help someone with depression to develop adaptive strategies to tackle the challenges inherent in managing difficulties in interpersonal relationships.

IPT is organized around four primary interpersonal focal areas:

+ difficulty adjusting to important and unwelcome change (role transition);
+ not getting on with someone who is important in your life (role dispute);
+ difficulty adjusting when someone close dies (grief);
+ difficulty making or keeping friends and close relationships (interpersonal sensitivity/deficits).

Goals are central to the therapy and are focused on the factors that maintain current depressive symptoms in one of these four focal areas. Reducing depressive symptoms and improving interpersonal relationships are common goals across all the IPT focal areas, in discussion with the person and they are personalized for each individual, through collaborative discussion. Unlike some other therapies, IPT does not set goals until the end of the assessment phase, typically around session 4 of 12-16 weekly sessions, with goals reflecting the collaboratively agreed focus of the intervention rather than directing the course of therapy from the outset.

How are goals conceptualized in IPT?

In session 1, the 'sick role' is agreed. This uses psychoeducation to help the person and their network to recognize the impact of depression and adjustments necessary to assist with recovery, for example by seeing friends regularly. This introduces the first general goal in IPT, to promote recovery, with the negotiated application of psychoeducation to initiate early change.

During the assessment phase, the therapy dyad collaboratively explore the impact of depression on current relationships. This bidirectional relationship between symptoms and relationships is used to frame a formulation of the current episode of depression in an interpersonal context. The goals are collaboratively selected to target the vulnerability and maintaining factors identified in the formulation and explicitly reflect the chosen focal area.

Each focal area has broad, overarching goals for example mourning the loss of the old role and exploring opportunities in the new role in role transitions, and these are then personalized to reflect the specific factors that are important for each person, for example find new ways to maintain contact with an absent parent when a family splits up or join a running club as a way to make friends after moving to a new area. Useful goals in IPT not only name the activity or change, for example join a running club, but also set out the reason why this would be helpful interpersonally, for example to make new friends and increase the amount of pleasure the person experiences. The formulation-based symptom and interpersonal objectives are made explicit.

How are goals used and monitored in IPT?

Clients are encouraged to refine and clarify their goals with input from their IPT therapist and 'goal buddies in their family and friends support team', who will help the person to achieve their objectives. Goals are written down and progress is rated on a 0-10 scale over the course of therapy. Progress towards these goals is frequently monitored and re-rated in subsequent sessions. Goal buddies may also be invited to rate progress towards goals during, and at the end of therapy. Inviting another perspective can provide invaluable opportunities for mentalizing between the person and their team members and ensures that the person's objectives are held in mind in the network as well as in the therapy room.

Some simple, general tips are offered to guide this process:

♦ Describe each goal in a single sentence to keep it simple.

♦ Don't aim for more than three goals to keep it manageable. Goals can be replaced later if good progress is achieved on the initial targets.

♦ Be specific not general and name the people being targeted, for example 'I will see my friend Joe once a week' rather than, 'I will do more'.

♦ Identify the change you will work towards and how this will contribute to improving symptoms and relationships.

♦ Write your goals down and go back to them regularly.

♦ Describe your goals to someone else to make sure they are clear and to ask how they can help.

♦ Focus on what you are going to do and not what other people need to do, for example 'I want my parents to listen to me' becomes 'I want to learn to communicate clearly and calmly'.

It is also often helpful to break goals down into short-, medium-, and long-term plans. Short-term goals are designed to build in an early experience of success by identifying objectives that are readily achievable in the first few weeks of therapy, for example telling team members about IPT and watching videos or reading relevant information together to help the person and the team understand depression, how it is treated, and what they can do. Examples of commonly used information and videos are available here:

♦ MindEd module on IPT-A
https://www.minded.org.uk/LearningContent/LaunchForGuestAccess/447810

♦ I had a black dog, his name was depression
https://www.youtube.com/watch?v=XiCrniLQGYc

♦ Living with a Black Dog
https://www.youtube.com/watch?v=2VRRx7Mtep8

- short film about three young people who have recovered from depression http://www.bbc.co.uk/education/clips/zxqcd2p

Medium-term goals are objectives to work towards over the course of therapy and will specifically reflect the focal area that has been chosen. These will significantly influence the choice of interventions over the remaining weeks of therapy.

Long-term goals are designed to conceptualize objectives that will be achieved after the therapy sessions have concluded but to which therapy will contribute, for example joining a social club during freshers' week for a young person who plans to go to college in the months following the end of therapy. By making these goals explicit at the outset the IPT therapist clearly communicates that the aim of therapy is not to fix everything and holds the reality of ending in focus for this time-limited therapy.

References and further reading

Additional details of the IPT-A approach and work with goals specifically can be found in:

Dietz, L., Weinberg, R. J., Brent, D. & Mufson, L. (2015). Family based interpersonal psychotherapy for depressed preadolescents: Examining efficacy and potential treatment mechanisms. *Journal of American Academy of Adolescent Psychiatry, 54*(3), 191–9.

Law, R. (2013). *Defeating Depression—Using the people in your life to open the door to recovery*. London: Constable and Robinson. https://www.littlebrown.co.uk/books/detail.page?isbn=9781849017121

Law, R. (2016). *Defeating Teenage Depression—Getting There Together*. London: Little Brown Books. https://www.littlebrown.co.uk/books/detail.page?isbn=9781472120250

Markowitz, J. C., & Weissman, M. M. (Eds.) (2012). *Casebook of Interpersonal Psychotherapy*. New York: Oxford University Press.

Mufson, L., Pollack Dorta, K., Moreau, D. & Weissman, M. M. (2004). *Interpersonal Psychotherapy for depressed adolescents* (2nd ed.). New York: Guilford Press.

Humanistic and existential therapy

Mick Cooper

Humanistic and existential therapies are a family of therapeutic approaches that aim to help clients 'actualize' their potential as human beings (Cain, Keenan, & Rubin, 2016). It includes person-centred, gestalt, and emotion-focused therapies; as well as the various schools of existential therapy, such as the meaning-centred and existential-phenomenological approaches. Existential and humanistic therapies are used with adults, young people, and children; primarily on a one-to-one basis, but also in groups.

Humanistic and existential therapies are based on the assumption that psychological difficulties emerge when people become estranged from their genuine human experiencing. To help clients establish a more 'authentic' way of being, humanistic and existential therapists primarily work in *relational* ways. Here, therapists strive to create a warm, empathic, and trustworthy therapeutic relationship in which clients can 'reconnect' with their actual subjective experiencing. Humanistic and existential therapists may also use a range of methods—such as 'two-chair work' and 'focusing'—to help clients connect more deeply with their authentic emotions, needs, and perceptions.

Traditionally, members of the humanistic and existential community have been wary of goal-oriented practices (e.g. Rowan, 2008). This is for a number of inter-related reasons, as discussed in the introduction to this book (Chapter 1). First, they can be seen as setting an agenda and direction for therapy, while many humanistic and existential practitioners prefer to work in 'non-directive' ways: allowing whatever emerges for the client, at whatever time, to become the therapeutic focus (e.g. Rogers, 1951). Second, goal-oriented practice may be seen as prioritising 'doing'—activity, behaviour, and striving—over a more 'natural' and 'authentic' state of 'being'. Third, it may be seen as putting expectations upon clients—that they should *achieve* something through therapy—rather than unconditionally accepting them for however they are. Fourth, there may be concerns that any goals set for therapy are more a reflection of the therapist's assumptions and agenda than the client's intrinsic, authentic needs and purposes. Finally, and closely related to this, verbally articulated goals—particularly as stated at the start of therapy—may be seen as representing only the client's conscious, surface-level, extrinsic wants; and not the deeper, intrinsic, organismic needs that, if fulfilled, will lead to a genuinely more fulfilling and satisfying life.

However, countering these arguments, there are ways in which a goal-focused practice can be seen as deeply compatible with an existential and humanistic approach. First, while some existential and humanistic writers, as indicated above, privilege being (i.e. experiencing) over doing (i.e. activity), there are many others who would consider 'doing' as fundamental to, and inseparable from, 'being'. For Heidegger (1996), for instance, the most influential of the existential philosophers, our being-in-the-world is always a doing: a 'caught up-ness' in undertakings and activities. More specifically, for both him and Sartre (1996), our being-in-the-world has a strongly future-oriented dimension. Writes Sartre, for instance, 'Man first of all is the being who hurls himself towards a future and who is conscious of imagining himself as being in the future' (p. 259). This is reflected in the humanistic view of people as agentic, intentional, and self-directed (e.g. Bohart & Tallman, 1999). From this perspective, then, it could be argued that goal-directed activity is intrinsic to human being, and that goal-setting is not an external imposition on clients, but a means of helping clients articulate something at the very essence of their existence.

Setting goals can also be seen as a means of empowering clients—which is at the heart of the humanistic agenda—helping them take a more active role in determining the nature and direction of the therapeutic work. Although there is the possibility that goals may reflect a therapist's agenda, this would not be considered competent goal-focused practice, as detailed in this book. Moreover, it would be naïve of therapists to assume that, by not setting goals with clients, their own agendas are thereby absent from the therapeutic process. Rather, therapists will inevitably enter into the therapeutic work with particular needs, expectations, and objectives—unconscious as well as conscious. Hence, explicitly agreeing goals with clients can be a means of ensuring that the clients' own goals take precedence. This is also about transparency—a keystone of humanistic and existential practice—whereby agendas and needs are talked about in an honest and upfront manner.

Given the concerns that have existed in the humanistic and existential field regarding goal-focused practices, a humanistic and existential approach to working with goals is only beginning to emerge (e.g. Cooper & McLeod, 2011). However, reflecting the values and practices of this approach (as discussed above), it emphasizes a number of different elements of goal-oriented work: many of which may be shared across practices. First, there is a strong emphasis on ensuring that goals emerge from the client, rather than from the therapist: a 'client-centred' approach. Second, there is a particular openness to clients modifying and adjusting their goals during the course of therapy. In addition, from this relatively 'non-directive' standpoint, goals would tend to be understood as approximate directions to which the client is oriented, rather than fixed and definitive objectives by which they will be judged.

A case example may help to illustrate this. At the start of the therapeutic work, Marek's goals were to understand how he felt towards his marriage, and to reduce anger and distrust towards his wife. However, over time, these evolved into finding himself again, and becoming more connected with what he wanted in life. Here, the therapist was supportive towards Marek in revising his goals, and offered him regular opportunities to revisit them, and to reflect on whether they still represented what he was most striving for. In addition, the goals were held fairly 'lightly' in the therapeutic work. So, for instance, although Marek was encouraged to rate his goals every week, if he went on to talk about other issues in the sessions, he was supported to do so rather than being drawn back to focus on his goals.

Although it is still at a nascent stage, a goal-oriented approach may have the potential to enhance and develop humanistic and existential practices. In addition, however, a goal-oriented practice may also have much to learn from humanistic and existential therapies. First, the concepts and ideas of existential writers, as introduced above, can provide a rich and powerful philosophical grounding on which to develop a goal-oriented understanding of human being. Second, developments in the meaning-centred therapies field (Vos, 2016) provide a range of new methods by which clients can be helped towards their goals and purposes. Furthermore, human and existential writings on the relationship and the introduction of new relational concepts, such as 'relational depth' (Mearns & Cooper, 2017), can help to ensure that a goal-focused practice always emerges from a warm, empathic, and collaborative therapeutic relationship.

Points for reflection

◆ Which therapies do you think goal-oriented practices are *most* compatible with? Which do you think they are *least* compatible with?

◆ To what extent do you think goal-oriented practices complement, or interfere with, your own therapeutic orientation?

References

Bohart, A. C., & Tallman, K. (1999). *How Clients Make Therapy Work: The Process of Active Self-Healing*. Washington: American Psychological Association.

Cain, D., Keenan, K., & Rubin, S. (Eds.). (2016). *Humanistic psychotherapies* (2nd ed.). Washington: APA.

Heidegger, M. (1996). *Being and Time* (J. Stambaugh, Trans.). Albany, NY: State University of New York Press.

Mearns, D., & Cooper, M. (2017). *Working at Relational Depth in Counselling and Psychotherapy* (2nd ed.). London: Sage.

Rogers, C. R. (1951). *Client-Centered Therapy*. Boston: Houghton and Mifflin.

Rowan, J. (2008). Goals. *BACP North London Magazine*(59), 7.

Sartre, J.-P. (1996). Existentialism. In L. Cahoone (Ed.), *From Modernism to Postmodernism: An Anthology* (pp. 259–65). Cambridge, MA: Blackwells Publishers Ltd.

Vos, J. (2016). Working with meaning in life in mental health care: a systematic literature review and meta-analyses of the practices and effectiveness of meaning-centered therapies. In P. Russo-Netzer, S. E. Schulenberg & A. Batthyany (Eds.), *To thrive, to cope, to understand—Meaning in positive and existential psychotherapy*. New York: Springer.

Chapter 10

Conclusion

Duncan Law and Mick Cooper

The analogy of travel is often applied to counselling and psychotherapy: therapy as a journey of discovery or a journey from one state of mind to another. So it is perhaps fitting that this conclusion was written as one of the authors travelled down the western coast of the Indian sub-continent from Mumbai to Kanyakumari, at the southernmost tip of India. Navigating the Indian transport system for a foreigner is not straightforward but, luckily, there was usually someone more than willing to offer help and guidance. Interestingly, the offers of help were most often instigated with the opening question: 'What do you want?' rather than the more travel context-specific question; 'Where do you want to go?'.

As a traveller, 'What do you want?' may be a more liberating and useful opening question than 'Where do you want to go?'. Depending on one's reasons for travelling, and the time and resource at one's disposal, having a fixed endpoint is not always important or desirable: some of life's greatest adventures come when one does not have a goal or destination in mind, but goes where the next train or bus takes you. 'What do you want?' leaves the options open to travel for discovery and exploration, or travel to a desired destination. Both are travel, but both have different aims and objectives and strategies to get what you want from the travelling. What is needed from the offer, 'What do you want?' and who is best placed to help you, is different depending on the aims of your journey.

So it is with psychotherapy and counselling. For some, the engagement with the work is to explore and discover, and they want help to facilitate the exploration. For others, they are clear where they want to go and want help and guidance to navigate how best to get there. Others may not have any answer (yet) to the question 'What do you want?' and may not even know if they want anything at all, and want help to see if they can find an answer to the question. All these reasons for entering into counselling or psychotherapy are valid and offering different types of therapeutic experiences depending on what clients want are equally valid too.

These different motivations for seeking, and offering, counselling and psychotherapy link with the debate around the use and usefulness of goals in therapy. If the client wants a journey of discovery—setting off on an adventure not knowing where they might end up—tight, fixed therapy goals might be seen to limit rather than widen their horizons. Setting a goal too early, or even having a destination goal at all, might limit the outcome of the journey. On the other hand, for those who have, or want, a clear destination, then having a shared agreement on the goals of the therapy is likely to be helpful and provide focus and a shared understanding of the work. And for those who do not yet know what they want, the focus of the work might be an exploration that leads to setting a goal—which may involve counselling as a vehicle, or may not. All these are a matter of personal preference and context and we must be careful not to make *a priori* judgements. It is as unhelpful to debate which is the 'best' therapeutic strategy as it is to debate which form of travel is the 'best'. The best kind of therapy (travel) is the one that best fits the needs and wishes and preferences and context of the client. But here is the crux of the matter: before therapists can offer the right kind of help or guidance or facilitation, they need to ask the client (perhaps not so bluntly): 'What do you want?'.

'What do you want?' is a deceptively simple question that draws on quite complex psychological processes and requires great therapeutic skills to help a client answer. But, from the perspective developed in this book, the client's answer to this question should set the overarching direction for the therapeutic process itself. Unless we know the client's reasons for embarking on a therapeutic journey, we cannot be as helpful as we or they might wish. How we help and how we understand the question, how we support and facilitate the client to find the answer that is right for them and the myriad potential answers to it, is the starting point for how we help and how we go on being helpful. This is about how we help the client start, and how we remain flexible and open to changes in the directions and reasons for travel, and how we seek to work to be as helpful as we can in joining the client on their journey. We may choose to call what the client wants: 'therapeutic goals', or we might just call it 'being helpful'. Furthermore, we may choose to make these goals more explicit in the therapy and call this 'goal-oriented practice', and we might even choose to use tools to track or score progress towards goals. The semantics are far less important than the importance of the processes we employ to help clients get to where they want to be.

So it is with this book: you will have had your reasons for reading it. You may have chosen to travel all the way through it, or to visit different chapters and not others. Some sections you may have liked and disliked more than others; some sections will have seemed familiar, perhaps even boring; other sections may have been challenging and uncomfortable; other sections may have been fascinating and enlightening. Whatever your reasons for engaging with it, we hope the journey was worthwhile and it has, even in some small way, helped you get to where you want to go.

We wish you all the best on your travels ...

Index

Note: Tables and figures are indicated by an italic *t* and *f* following the page number.